Acupuncture Information Manual

(AIM)

An Evidence-Based Resource Manual on the Use of Acupuncture for Over 40 Common Medical Conditions

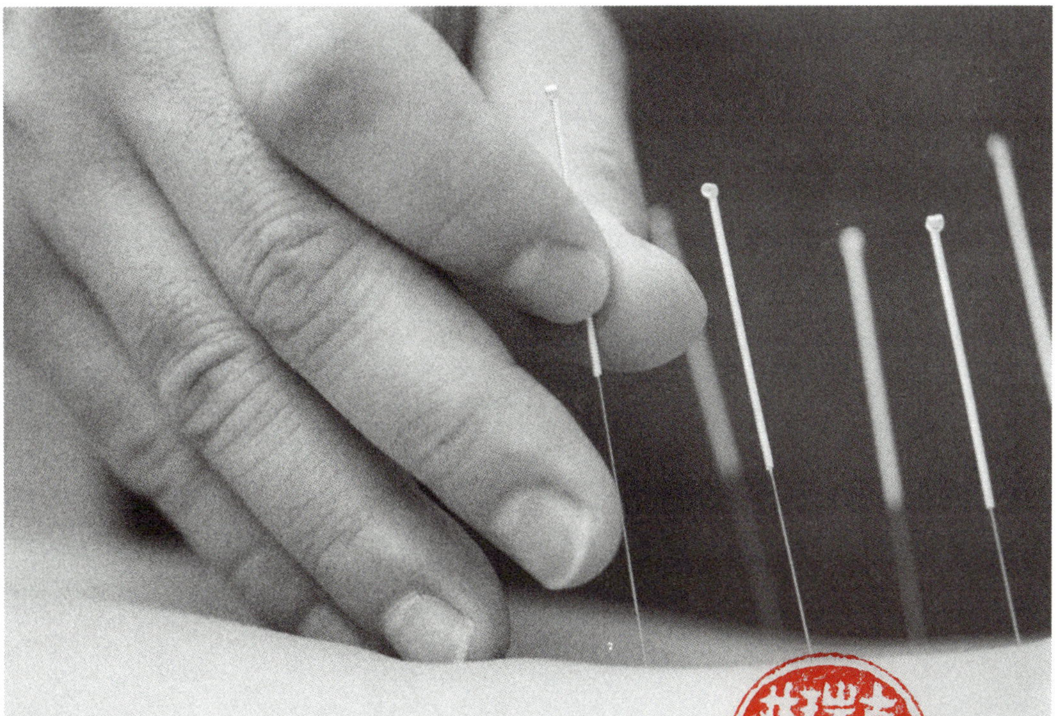

Eric P. Hunstad, L.Ac

www.AcupunctureInformationManual.com

First Edition

Published by Eric P. Hunstad

ISBN-13: 978-0-692-98980-7

Table of Contents

Part II- What Conditions Can Acupuncture Improve?

About the Author

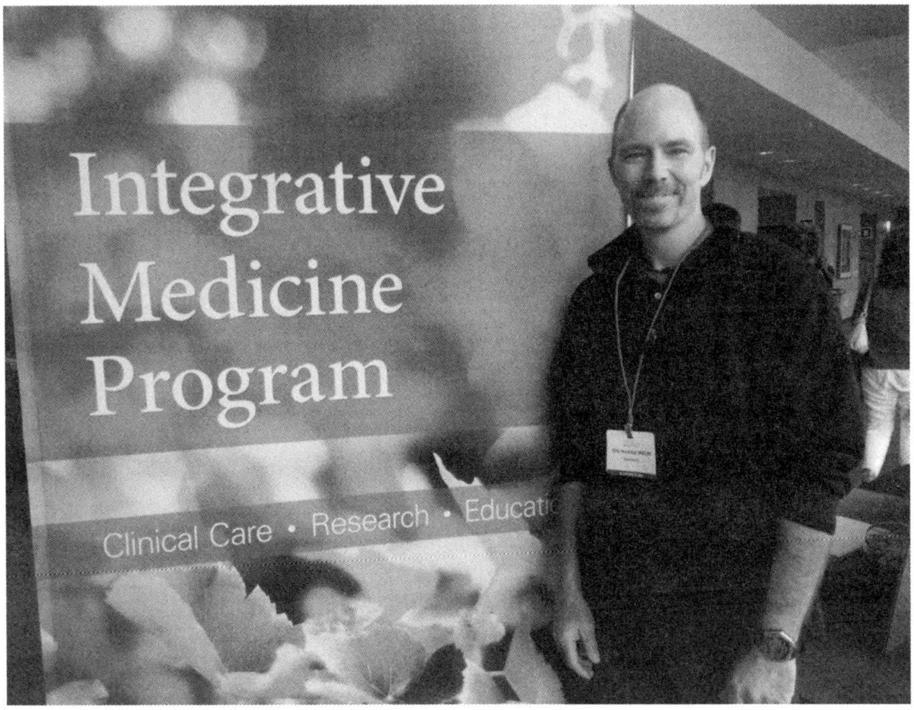

Eric P. Hunstad has a bachelor's degree in Psychology (graduated *cum laude* from the University of Central Florida), a bachelor's degree in Health Science, as well as a master's degree in Acupuncture and Oriental Medicine from the Florida College of Integrative Medicine. He is a licensed acupuncturist with a busy practice in Titusville, Florida.

www.TitusvilleAcupuncture.com

He also studied Chinese martial arts for over 25 years and is a certified instructor in the Three Treasures system of kung fu, and has extensive training in qi gong and Yang and Chen style taijiquan. He is the author of **"Old School Kung Fu"** which is available at **www.OldSchoolKungFuNow.com** .

Introduction

Acupuncture is one component of Traditional Chinese Medicine, and Chinese martial arts are deeply rooted in Traditional Chinese Medicine. It is through Chinese martial arts that I was exposed to the genius, the beauty, and the effectiveness of Traditional Chinese Medicine. I was raised in a medical family, but early on I realized that there were limitations in medical standards of care. In my early teens, I started training in kung fu, and my teacher was also a doctor of Traditional Chinese Medicine. He placed a strong emphasis on health and included health education into our training. He also would treat us for any injuries we sustained or if any health issues came up. From my own personal experience, I learned that Traditional Chinese Medicine could work wonders.

I knew from a young age that I wanted to help people for a living, and I also had a personal interest in psychology. After high school, I decided to get a degree in psychology with the intention of eventually obtaining a PhD. After graduating from the University of Central Florida with a bachelor's degree in psychology, I decided to get some work experience to help me decide what area I wanted to specialize in and assist me in becoming accepted into a post graduate psychology program.

I got a job at a mental health organization in central Florida and worked in their residential program working primary with schizophrenic patients. One year turned into several, as I kept getting promoted within the company and the work was fascinating. I continued to train in Chinese martial arts, and obtained my Sifu (instructor) level certification. After five years of working in mental health I had a moment of clarity and realized that I wanted to go "all in" with Traditional Chinese Medicine, so I abandoned my goal of obtaining a PhD in psychology and instead pursued a master's degree in acupuncture and Oriental medicine. I graduated from the Florida College of Integrative Medicine in 2003, passed the national NCCAOM board exam, and became a licensed acupuncturist.

Over the years, while working as an acupuncturist, I would constantly review the published medical research on acupuncture, and became somewhat of a "collector" of research studies. In the beginning, there were very few published studies, and the ones that were available were often low quality. But eventually that started to change and today there is a wealth of information regarding the effects of acupuncture on many medical conditions.

However, the information is not getting out to those who need it the most. The medical community often ignores these studies, while many acupuncturists are not even aware that they exist. Further, the patients interested in improving their health have no idea what the current research shows and unfortunately depend on internet searches to obtain information in order to make a decision on whether or not they should try acupuncture for their particular condition.

> "Reducing medical information to basic principles is like collecting items in a bag. When the bag is full but not bound, the information spills out and is lost."- **Yellow Emperor, Nan Jing Ling Shu 48 Obeying the Taboos**

It is my sincere intention to follow in the footsteps of the famous Yellow Emperor of ancient China and compile modern acupuncture evidence-based research into a format that gets the information to those that need it. With over one hundred referenced medical studies, the **Acupuncture Information Manual (AIM)** is a valuable resource for:

- Patients
- Medical Doctors and other Medical Professionals
- Licensed Acupuncturists

Patients can benefit from the wealth of information regarding how acupuncture can be explained by biomedical science, and they can also benefit from discovering the latest evidence-based research regarding how acupuncture can improve specific medical conditions which affect themselves or someone they love.

Medical Doctors and other Medical Professionals can benefit by reviewing the latest evidence-based research and learning that acupuncture is a safe and effective treatment option with scientific and clinical foundations in modern biomedicine. They can then use that information to make appropriate referrals and have confidence in those referrals.

Licensed Acupuncturists can benefit from discovering the latest evidence-based research regarding how acupuncture can improve specific medical conditions in order to help their patients. In addition, the manual can be used as an excellent patient education resource, thereby improving patient compliance and patient referrals.

It is also my hope that this manual will inspire others to continue to raise awareness of the efficacy of this incredible medicine, and to put acupuncture where it belongs- as a safe and effective treatment option for many modern healthcare conditions.

Eric P. Hunstad, L.Ac

November, 2017

Part I:

Acupuncture Explained

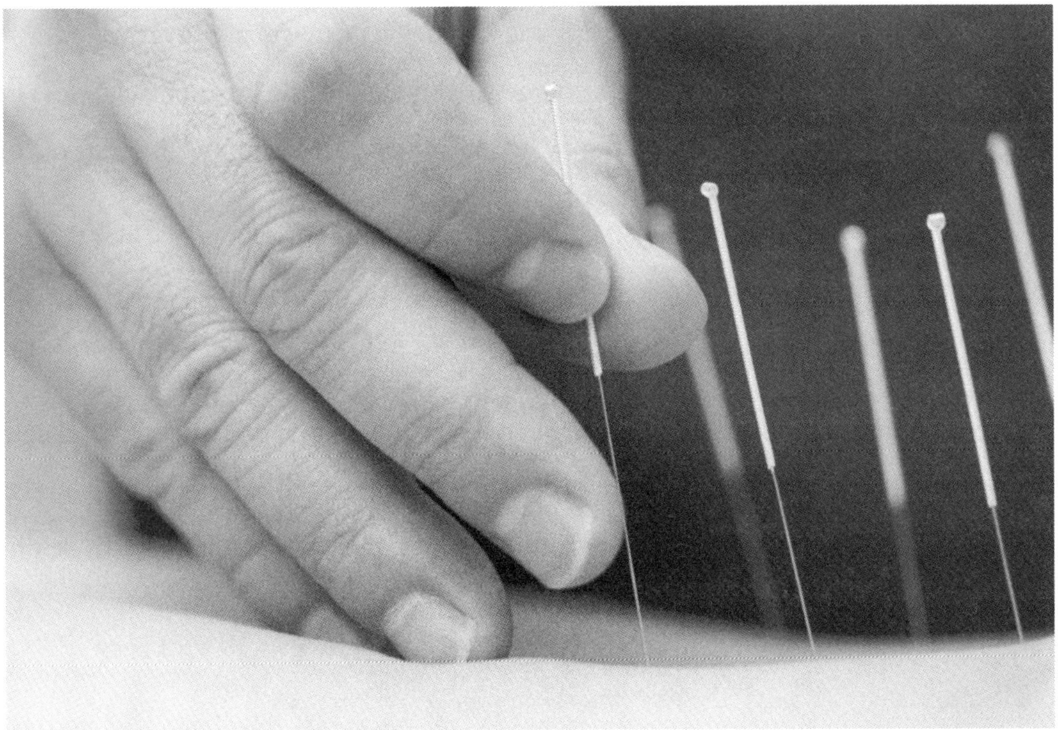

What is "Acupuncture"?

Acupuncture is the practice of placing small, specially designed, **surgical stainless steel** needles (called **"filiform"** needles) into various places in the body in order to promote healing. The special areas where these needles are placed are called "acupuncture points". These acupuncture points are linked together in pathways called "meridians".

Acupuncture is one part of **Traditional Chinese Medicine (TCM),** which has been in practice for over 2,500 years. Just the fact that it has survived for so long is evidence of its value as a healing art (if it didn't have value something else would have replaced it).

> **"Acupuncture hacks into the systems that monitor and adjust the body's own resources, thus facilitating self-healing and symptom management"- Acupuncture Now Foundation**

A quick Google search will provide lots of information regarding acupuncture. But the vast majority of it generally boils down to two primary schools of thought. On one side, there is the belief by traditionalists that acupuncture is the manipulation of mystical energy called “Chi” or “Qi”. They feel qi is balanced by inserting a uniquely designed needle into special points in the body in order to promote health and healing by increasing or decreasing the amount of “qi” in the “meridians”.

On the other side, there is a belief by skeptics that acupuncture is nothing more than an elaborate and potentially expensive placebo.

Luckily the explosion in acupuncture research over the last 20 years has generated a wealth of scientific information regarding acupuncture (if you know where to find it) and a new school of thought is emerging: **Acupuncture is a safe and effective treatment option with scientific and clinical foundations in modern biomedicine.**

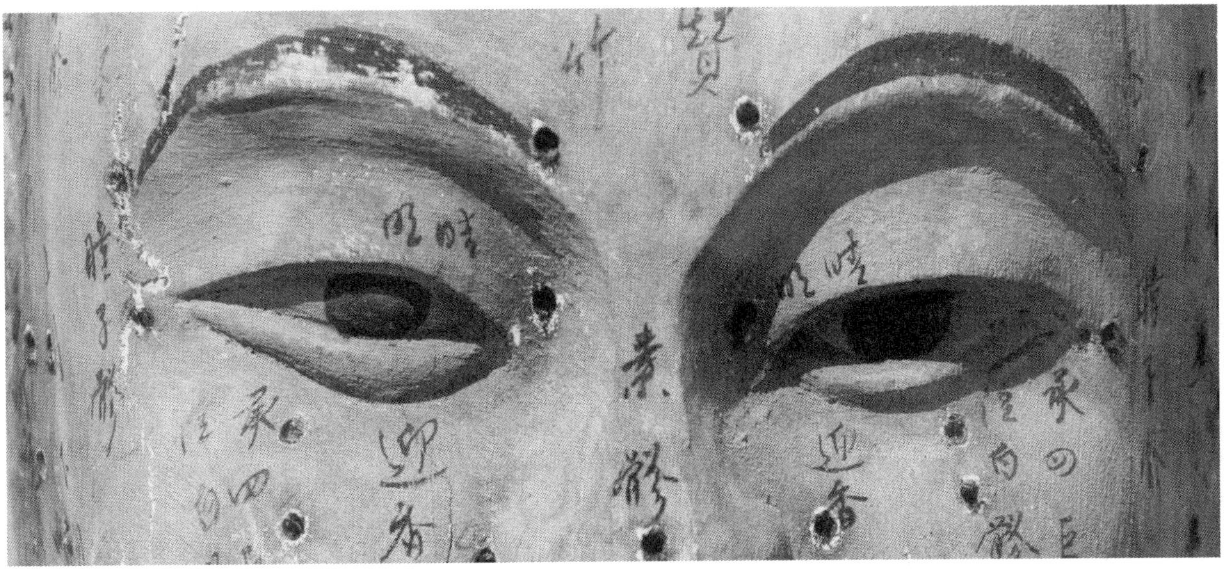

What are "Acupuncture Points"?

In Traditional Chinese Medicine, acupuncture points are considered to be special areas of the body which can be stimulated to "balance the body's energies".

But what are acupuncture points from a modern **medical perspective**? Pioneering research to investigate the unique anatomical properties of acupuncture points, also known as "**acupoints**", systematically began in 1959. Since then, many **researchers** have attempted to answer the question from a **biomedical** perspective.

Newer studies have shown that 323 out of 324 acupoints are associated with nerves, and that acupoints represent "**unique neuroanatomical targets**". This suggests that the ancient acupuncturists had a **deep understanding** of the **nervous system** (**"The Point of Acupuncture",** ***Medical Acupuncture*** **V27, No. 2, April 2015).**

Modern science shows that acupuncture points are simply special areas of the body that possess unique physical and biological properties. These special properties can be utilized to assist the body in self-regulating and to accelerate healing.

Dive Deeper into Biomedicine- Acupoint Properties

Anatomical studies have identified that the number of **nerve fibers/trunks**, **blood vessels**, **hair follicles**, and **sweat glands** are enhanced over acupoints compared to their adjacent control areas.

Also, studies have demonstrated that **nitric oxide synthases (NOS)** protein levels and **nitric oxide (NO)** contents are **consistently higher** in skin regions containing acupoints compared to control tissues in rats **("Enhanced Nitric Oxide Concentrations and Expression of Nitric Oxide Synthase in Acupuncture Points/Meridians",** ***J Complement Med*** **2003 Apr; 9(2):207-215). https://www.ncbi.nlm.nih.gov/pubmed/12804074**

This is important because nitric oxide plays a critical role in blood pressure and circulation. Interestingly, gender and race do not influence NO release over the acupoints, but age and obesity do influence it **("Influence of Age, Gender, and Race on Nitric Oxide Release Over Acupuncture Points-Meridians",** ***Sci Rep*** **2015; 5: 17547). https://www.ncbi.nlm.nih.gov/pmc/articles/PMC4664911/**

In addition, acupuncture points have demonstrated **"neuronal specificity",** meaning that simulating an acupuncture point will have **specific effects** over stimulating non-acupuncture points (called "**sham points**" in research studies) located in the same spinal segment. In other words, stimulating an acupoint produces specific effects compared to stimulating anywhere else in the body. This is referred to as "**acupoint specificity**".

In an interesting fMRI study, electro-acupuncture was used to stimulate two different points, both located in the L5 spinal segment. The actual acupoint (left *Yanglingquan* GB34) was shown to have specific effects more related to motor function, which is exactly what the point is commonly used to treat.

Dive Deeper into Biomedicine- Acupoint Properties Con't.

The researchers concluded "The results of this study provide **neurobiological evidence** for the existence of acupoint specificity" **("An fMRI Study of Neuronal Specificity of an Acupoint: Electro-Acupuncture Stimulation of Yanglingquan (GB34) and its Sham Point",** ***Neurosci Lett*** **2009 Oct 16; 464(1): 1-5). https://www.ncbi.nlm.nih.gov/pubmed/19666085**

Finally, acupuncture can have **different effects** on the **brain** depending on which **side** of the **body** the acupoint is stimulated on. In an interesting fMRI study, stimulating acupoint *Yanglingquan* GB34 on the right leg had different effects on the brain than when it was stimulated on the left leg **("Ipsilateral Putamen and Insula Activation by Both Left and Right GB34 Acupuncture Stimulation: An fMRI Study on Healthy Participants",** ***Evid Based Comp and Altern Med,*** **V. 2016, article ID 4173185).**
https://www.hindawi.com/journals/ecam/2016/4173185/

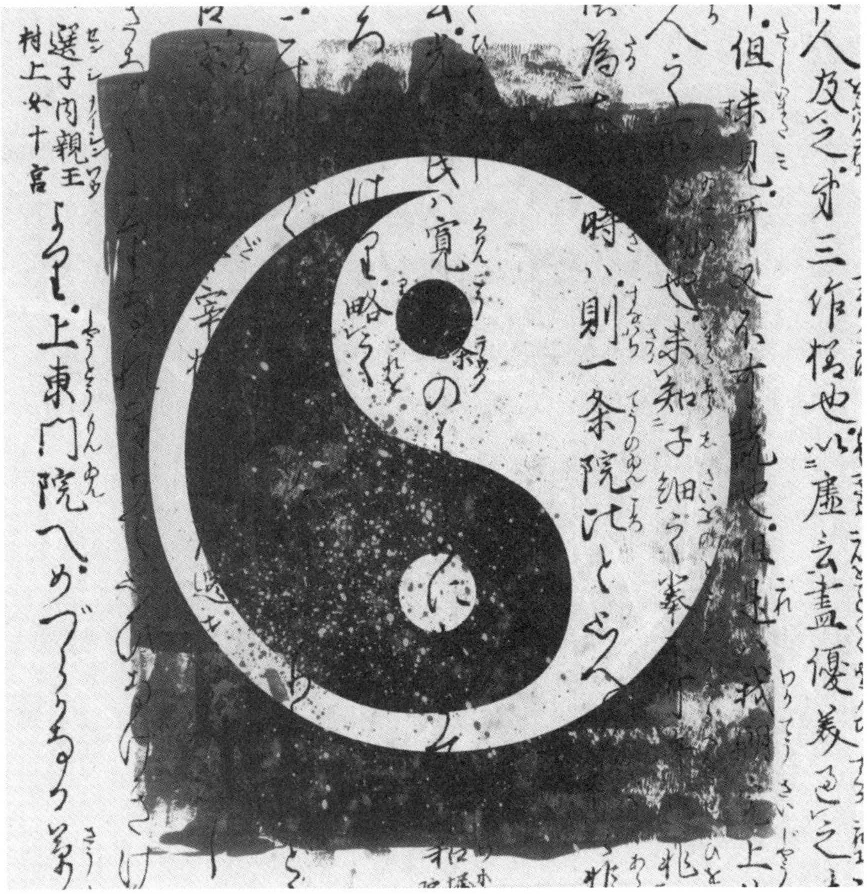

What is "Qi"?

In Traditional Chinese Medicine, qi is explained as an invisible energy which circulates throughout the body. It is considered the **"life force"** and it is the foundation of traditional acupuncture. Because there is currently no way to directly measure qi, skeptics feel that it doesn't exist.

But the Chinese character for what the ancients called qi has **many** meanings, depending on **context** in which it's written. One **general** meaning is "**the function of**", so when they say "the kidney qi is weak", what they are saying is that the function of the kidney system is weak, which could also be referred to as early stage renal failure.

There are other general meanings of the word qi as well that can be confirmed by biomedicine. For example, the ancient Chinese knew that some **invisible pathogen** could enter the body through the nose and throat and make a person sick. They called this "evil qi invading the body", while today we refer to this as a **viral** or **bacterial infection.** Interestingly, the **herbs** they prescribed to expel the "evil qi" just happen to have **antibiotic** and **antiviral** properties.

The Traditional Chinese Medicine concept of "qi" is complex and there are many explanations for it, from the relatively simple **("nerve impulse")** to the more complex **("intracellular communication system")**, to the abstract **("metaphysical energy")**.

Dive Deeper into Biomedicine- Medical Explanations for the Concepts of Qi

As stated earlier, the concept of "qi" has many interpretations, depending on the context in which it's written. There are many **medical explanations** for the many meanings of "qi":

Oxygen Metabolism: The term "qi" can refer to the metabolism of oxygen in the body, and the "qi-blood" that circulates through the "meridians" has been shown to correlate to the movement of oxygenated blood through the vascular system **("Oxygen and Meridian Qi", *Zhongguo Zhen Jiu* 2012 Feb; 32(2): 183-6).**
https://www.ncbi.nlm.nih.gov/pubmed/22493934

Nerve impulse: During treatments, acupuncturists attempt to elicit the "**Qi sensation**" (called "**de qi**" in Chinese, meaning "**the arrival of qi").** This refers to the various feelings the patient experiences during the manipulation of the needle, including heaviness, dull ache, heat, etc.

Biomedically speaking, this "qi sensation" refers to the **depolarization** of the **peripheral nerve** via **mechanical transduction** achieved by **needle manipulation** at the correct acupoint location **("The Point of Acupuncture", *Medical Acupuncture*, V27, No.2, April 2015)**. Traditional acupuncture texts emphasize that "de qi" must be obtained in order to have clinical success in healing a patient.

Dive Deeper into Biomedicine- Medical Explanations for the Concepts of Qi Con't.

Using modern neuroscience, we now know which **specific nerve fibers** fire to cause each specific "qi sensation". For example, "**heaviness**" is caused by stimulation of **A-delta** and **III muscle fibers,** while "**heat**" is caused by stimulation of **C-fiber** and **IV muscle fibers**.

Cellular energy: The term "qi" can also relate to **chemical/cellular processes** in the body. For example, **oxygen metabolism** and **adenosine triphosphate (ATP)** production occur at a **cellular** level. ATP is a complex organic chemical that supplies large amounts of energy to cells for various biochemical processes, including muscle contraction and sugar metabolism. It is also a precursor to DNA and RNA. When an acupuncture needle is inserted into an area of highly innervated tissue ("acupuncture point"), local cells trigger the release of energy in the form of ATP (see **"Acupuncture Affects the Local Tissue"**).

Increased chemical communication via signaling molecules: There is a hypothesis that "qi" involves **signaling molecules** which travel via an **intercellular communication system**, and acupuncture at specific points enhances this communication system. **Nitric oxide (NO)** has been proposed to be one such signaling molecule **("Intercellular Communication, NO and the Biology of Chinese Medicine",** ***Cell Communication and Signaling,*** **2005 3:8). https://biosignaling.biomedcentral.com/articles/10.1186/1478-811X-3-8**

Nitric oxide regulates blood pressure, contributes to the immune response, controls neurotransmission and participates in **cell differentiation** and many more physiological functions.

As stated earlier, studies have demonstrated that **nitric oxide synthases (NOS)** protein levels and **nitric oxide (NO)** contents are **consistently higher** in skin regions containing acupoints compared to control tissues in rats **("Enhanced Nitric Oxide Concentrations and Expression of Nitric Oxide Synthase in Acupuncture Points/Meridians",** ***J Complement Med*** **2003 Apr; 9 (2):207-215). https://www.ncbi.nlm.nih.gov/pubmed/12804074**

Dive Deeper into Biomedicine- Medical Explanations for the Concepts of Qi Con't.

Other studies have shown that acupuncture increases the amount of NO in the peripheral blood **("Effects of Warm Needling at *Zusanli* (ST36) on NO and IL-2 Levels in Middle Aged and Old People", *J Tradit Chin Med,* 2003 Jun; 23(2):127-128). https://www.ncbi.nlm.nih.gov/pubmed/12875077**

Interestingly, it has been shown that gender and race do not influence NO release over the acupoints, but age and obesity do influence it **("Influence of Age, Gender, and Race on Nitric Oxide Release Over Acupuncture Points-Meridians", *Sci Rep* 2015; 5: 17547). https://www.ncbi.nlm.nih.gov/pmc/articles/PMC4664911/**

This fits the hypothesis that qi is a signaling molecule because traditionally qi is also thought to be reduced with age and obesity, but not with gender or race.

Traditional concept of "excess" or "deficient" qi: One of the most amazing things about acupuncture is its ability to promote the **self-regulation** in the body. Sometimes there is too much of a good thing (in Traditional Chinese Medicine terms, this is referred to as an "**excess**" condition).

In one study, **nitric oxide (NO)** levels were found to be **55% higher** in **migraine patients** compared to a control group. After **one** acupuncture treatment, migraine patients' NO levels **dropped 4.86%,** but after **five** acupuncture treatments, the NO levels of the migraine patients **dropped 30.63%** (bringing levels closer to **normal levels**).

This not only shows that acupuncture promotes **self-regulation** in the body, but it also shows the **cumulative effect** of acupuncture treatments **("The Impact of Acupuncture Treatment on Nitric Oxide (NO) in Migraine Patients", *Acupunct Electrother Res,* 2014; 39(3-4):275-83). https://www.ncbi.nlm.nih.gov/pubmed/25693309**

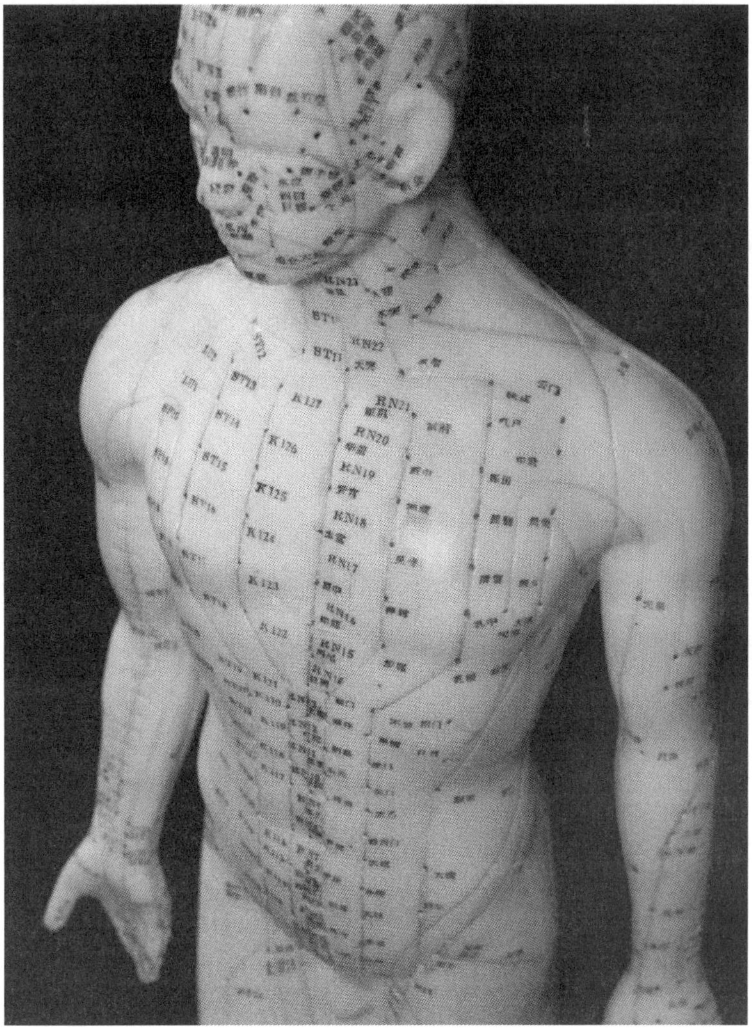

What are "Meridians"?

In **Traditional Chinese Medicine**, meridians are traditionally thought to be **invisible channels** that carry "qi" energy to nourish the entire body. Any disruption in this transportation system results in a reduction in the health of the body. The acupuncture points are located along these pathways or channels. Inserting an acupuncture needle into an acupoint is **traditionally** thought to be like turning a valve in order to either reduce or increase the amount of qi flowing through the channel.

The meridians can also be thought of as an ancient **mapping system** of the body, similar to the longitude and latitude lines on a globe. This assists with communication among acupuncturists (who were the leading medical providers along with herbalists at the time Traditional Chinese Medicine flourished). When an acupuncturists says a patient has pain at right *Quchi* (LI11), every other acupuncturist knows they are referring to the area of the right lateral epicondyle of the humerus (the area associated with tennis elbow). This enabled acupuncturists to communicate precisely (not to mention it makes modern acupuncturists SOAP notes much simpler!).

Dive Deeper into Biomedicine- Medical Theories of Meridians

The concept of "**meridians**" has been subject to **considerable research** over the years. Recently, one researcher summed up the current understanding of "meridians", stating "Despite numerous research endeavors with **modern science** on the meridian system, only the **phenomena** of meridians has been **confirmed**, and the structure, biomolecules, and functions of the pathways, especially the relationship between the somatic meridian and the internal organs, still remain unclear" **(*Scientific Reports,* December 2015).**

A brief overview of the leading theories of what the meridians actually are from a medical perspective:

Theory: Meridians are" Connective Tissue Planes"

There is some evidence that the meridians represent a previously unknown **connective tissue matrix** in the body. An interesting study demonstrating the map of a meridian pathway involved the injection of **Technitium99,** a radioactive tracer, into both true and sham acupuncture points. The scan of the injection sites showed **random diffusion** of the tracer around the sham points, but rapid **progression** of the tracer **along the meridian** at a rate that was inconsistent with either lymphatic/vascular flow or nerve conduction **(Nuclear Medicine Investigation of Transmission of Acupuncture Information, *Acupuncture in Medicine, BMJ,* V11 no. 1, May 1993). http://aim.bmj.com/content/11/1/22**

Dive Deeper into Biomedicine- Medical Theories of Meridians Con't.

Other studies which support this theory include:

"Relationship of Acupuncture Points and Meridians to Connective Tissue Planes", ***Anat Rec*** **2002 Dec 15; 269(6):257-265 https://www.ncbi.nlm.nih.gov/pubmed/12467083,**

"Connective Tissue: A Body-Wide Signaling Network?", ***Med Hypothesis*** **2006;66(6):1074-7 https://www.ncbi.nlm.nih.gov/pubmed/16483726**

"Tracing Mercox Injected at Acupuncture Points Under the Protocol of Partial Body Macerations in Mice" ***Journal of Acupuncture and Meridian Studies*****, V8, Issue 6, Dec 2015 pp. 314-320 http://www.sciencedirect.com/science/article/pii/S2005290115001521**

Theory: Meridians are "Migration Channels of Interstitial Fluid"

This theory is similar to the **Connective Tissue Planes Theory** but instead of connective tissue, it is theorized that meridians are **migration channels** of **interstitial fluid ("Visualized Regional Hypodermic Migration Channels of Interstitial Fluid in Human Beings: Are These Ancient Meridians?",** ***J Altern Complement Med.*** **2008 Jul; 14(6): 621-8). https://www.ncbi.nlm.nih.gov/pubmed/18684070**

Theory: Meridians are "Peripheral Nerve Pathways of the Central Nervous System".

This theory (called the **"Neural Hypothesis"**) has the **strongest evidence base**, and it is becoming clear that **the peripheral nervous system is the true foundation of the meridian system.**

Leading researchers state:

"Although there have been numerous theories concerning meridians and acupoints, we believe that the **peripheral nervous system** forms the main basis of acupoints as well as **afferent** and **efferent pathways** of the **acupuncture signals**" **(Acupuncture Therapy for Neurological Diseases, 2010 pg 32-80). https://link.springer.com/chapter/10.1007%2F978-3-642-10857-0_2**

Dive Deeper into Biomedicine- Medical Theories of Meridians Con't.

"The **Neural Hypothesis** is seen as the most **logical** and **consistent** explanation for the action of acupuncture" **("Defining Meridians: A Modern basis for Understanding",** ***J Acupunct Meridian Stud*** **2010; 3(2): 67-74).**
http://www.sciencedirect.com/science/article/pii/S2005290110600143

"The evidence suggests that acupuncture classic texts share the **same foundation** in **anatomy** and **physiology** as **current biomedicine,** only they use a **different language**, **imager**y, and **philosophy** to describe the same **peripheral nervous system**" **(The Point of Acupuncture,** ***Medical Acupuncture,*** **V27, No.2, April 2015).**

The mammoth work of **Will Chapple** at the **World Medicine Institute** supports this concept, and is a **great resource** for those wishing to learn the neuroanatomy of the acupuncture points and meridians **("Proposed Catalog of the Neuroanatomy and the Stratified Anatomy for the 361 Acupuncture Points of 14 Channels"** ***Journal of Acupuncture and Meridian Studies,*** **V6, Issue 5, Oct 2013, PP 270-274).**
http://www.sciencedirect.com/science/article/pii/S2005290113000022

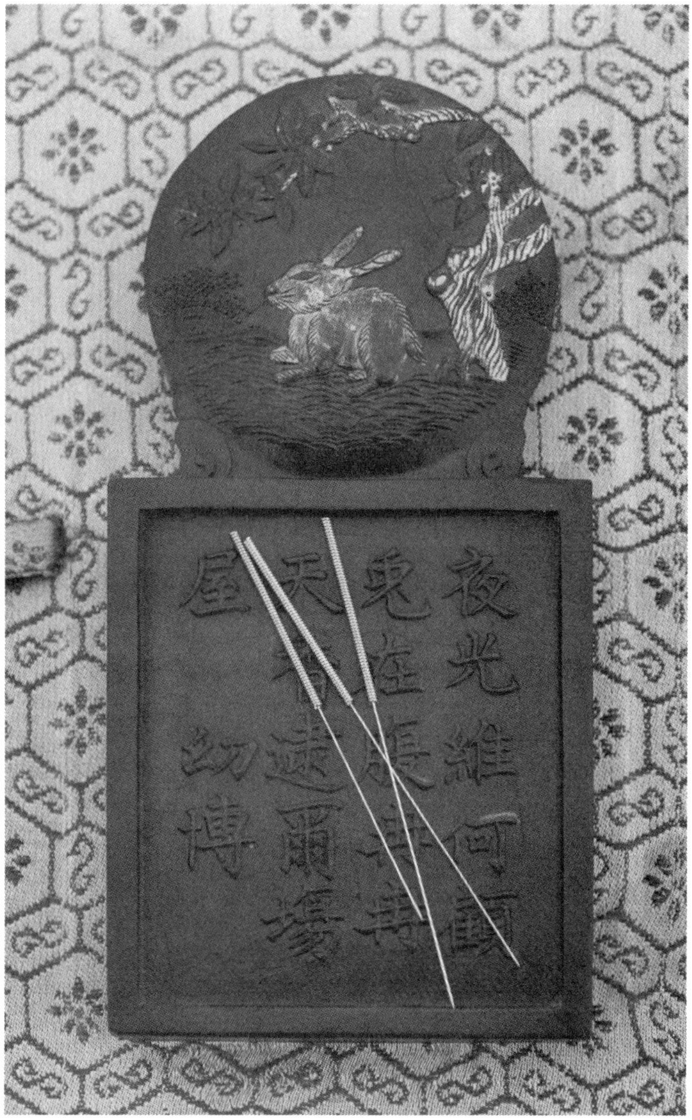

How Does Acupuncture Work?

> **"It is no longer possible to say that the effectiveness of acupuncture is because of the placebo effect, or that it is useful only for musculoskeletal pain" - The Acupuncture Evidence Project (www.acupuncture.org.au).**

Early acupuncture research focused on pain, and it was soon discovered that acupuncture triggers the release of **opioid peptides** (natural pain killers) in the central nervous system

("Acupuncture in Heroin Addicts: Changes in Met-Enkephalin and Beta-Endorphin in Blood and Cerebrospinal Fluid", *Lancet* 1979; 2 (8139):380-383).

Modern research shows that acupuncture achieves its many effects through very **complex physiological mechanisms.** But in a nutshell, studies show that inserting acupuncture needles into areas of **highly innervated tissue** (aka "acupuncture points") "triggers local, segmental, and heterosegmental effects; and influences, via reflex mechanisms, the **autonomic nervous system (ANS),** the motor pathways of the nervous system, and the immune and endocrine systems" **("Acupuncture- A Biomedical Information Therapy", *Medical Acupuncture* V28, number 6, 2016).**

Further, **electro-acupuncture** (the process of adding electrical stimulation to the acupuncture needles) can even influence the production of **mesenchymal stem cells (*Stem Cell* 2017: 35; 1303-1315) https://www.sciencedaily.com/releases/2017/03/170316174225.htm** and antioxidants **("The Antioxidative Effect of Electro-Acupuncture in a Mouse Model of Parkinson's Disease", *PLOS* May 23, 2011). https://doi.org/10.1371/journal.pone.0019790**

But to fully understand the incredible **complexity** of how acupuncture works (scientifically called acupuncture's **"mechanisms of action"**), is it best to look at the **specific effects** of acupuncture on the **different aspects** of the **body**.

Acupuncture Affects the Local Tissue

When an acupuncture needle is inserted into the body at specific areas of **nerve-rich tissue** (acupuncture points), a **complex chain reaction** occurs. For starters, local tissue cells trigger the release of energy in the form of **adenosine triphosphate,** commonly referred to as **"ATP"** (as stated before, this may be an example of the Traditional Chinese Medicine concept of increasing the "qi").

Acupuncture causes a tiny amount of "trauma" at just the right spot, which stimulates many survival mechanisms of the body.

ATP is a **complex organic chemical** that supplies large amounts of energy to cells for various biochemical processes, including **muscle contraction** and **sugar metabolism.** It is also a precursor to **DNA** and **RNA.** ATP is broken down to **adenosine** which is then taken up into the cells. Adenosine has a local anesthetic effect, and has also been shown to help **cartilage repair** and slow the progression of arthritis **("Endogenous Adenosine Maintains Cartilage Homeostasis and Inhibits Osteoarthritis Progression",** ***Nature Communications,*** **Sept. 7, 2016). http://www.nature.com/articles/ncomms15019**

Further, the local nerves fire (called an **"axon reflex"**) and signal the body to release a wide variety of **endogenous chemicals**, including red blood cells, white blood cells, histamines, and other complex substances and **biochemicals** which provide feedback to the brain and promote local healing.

Dive Deeper into Biomedicine- Acupuncture's Local Effects

When a needle is inserted into the body tissue, there is a **mechanistic deformation** of the local tissue. In response to this, cells generate cascades of **cellular** and **molecular events,** including cytoskeletal reorganization, cell contraction and migration, autocrine release of growth factors, and activation of intracellular signaling pathways and of nuclear binding proteins that promote the transcription of specific genes.

All of this leads to changes in the extracellular milieu surrounding needled tissues and finally promotes local healing. These effects may expand to distant connective tissue to spread the healing process with long term effects **("Science-based Mechanisms to Explain the Action of Acupuncture", *Journ of the Assoc of Trad Chin Med* (UK), V17, No. 2).** **http://noelravi.ee/wp-content/uploads/2015/07/Science-based-Mechanisms-to-Explain-the-Action-of-Acupuncture-2010.pdf**

There is also evidence of more complex, **morphologically verifiable** effects of acupuncture on fibroblasts, collagen fibers, and fascia, which are considered important because of their influence on the elasticity and mechanical characteristics of the connective tissue **("Acupuncture- A Biomedical Information Therapy", *Medical Acupuncture,* V28, Number 6, 2016).**

Acupuncture Affects Spinal Segments That Innervate Muscles, Organs, and Tissues

The **nervous system** consists of the brain, spinal cord, sensory organs, and all of the nerves that connect these organs with the rest of the body. The brain is the master controller, with the spinal cord connecting the brain to the nerves. The brain is protected by bone (the skull) and so is the spinal cord (protected by the flexible vertebra).

The nerves come out of the spinal cord at the nerve root, and there are nerve roots at each vertebral level of the spine. The nerves that exit the spine at each level go to various places, and innervate specific muscles, organs, and tissues.

The area where the nerve enters the spinal canal is called the **dorsal horn.** Bundles of nerves enter the dorsal horn at the **same level**, and if you can suppress the activity of the dorsal horn at a specific level, you affect both **somatic** (muscle) and **viscera**l (organ) nerves that converge at the dorsal horn at the same **neurotract**.

Placing an acupuncture needle into **highly innervated tissue** near a nerve root (aka "acupuncture point") produces a **complex series** of **neurotransmissions** (involving several types of nerve fibers) which results in effecting all nerve fibers at that level of the dorsal horn.

This means that placing an acupuncture needle near a nerve root at a particular level of the spine can affect both the <u>muscles</u> and <u>organs</u> that are innervated at the same spinal level.

Dive Deeper into Biomedicine- Somatotopic Organization of Acupoints

Acupuncture points located in the **same region** can have **different effects**, even though they are innervated at the same spinal segment. This is because a **"somatotopic"** organization (a point-for-point correspondence of an area of the body to a specific point on the central nervous system) has been demonstrated which may explain why not every acupuncture point located in the same dermatome is equally suited for producing a therapeutic effect **("Acupuncture- A Biomedical Information Therapy",** ***Medical Acupuncture,*** **V28, Number 6, 2016).**

Acupuncture Affects the Production of Endogenous Chemicals

Endogenous chemicals are chemicals that are made by the human body naturally. Early studies on acupuncture in the 1970's showed that acupuncture stimulated the release of **endogenous opiates** (natural pain killers). Newer studies have also shown acupuncture increases the neurotransmitters **serotonin** and **dopamine** as well. The latest studies have focused on **electro-acupuncture,** and what specific hertz and amperages produce specific neurotransmitters in the brain, allowing for a much more **targeted approach** to pain and other disorders.

Further, evidence is emerging that electro-acupuncture (at the correct hertz and amperage) can increase the effectiveness of **pain medication** allowing for a **lower dosage** and therefore **fewer side effects**.

Dive Deeper into Biomedicine- Adenosine

An interesting animal study demonstrated that acupuncture stimulates the release of **endogenous adenosine**, and that after 30 minutes of acupuncture, concentrations of adenosine had risen to a level **24 times** greater than its baseline levels **("The Secret Behind Acupuncture", *Science Illustrated*, July/August 2011).**

Adenosine is widely found in nature and plays an important role in biochemical processes, such as **energy** transfer-as **adenosine triphosphate (ATP)** and **adenosine diphosphate (ADP)**, as well as in signal transduction as cyclic **adenosine monophosphate (cAMP)**. It is a **neuromodulator** and it's believed to play a role in promoting sleep and suppressing arousal. Adenosine also plays a role in regulation of blood flow to various organs through **vasodilation**.

Dive Deeper into Biomedicine- Adenosine Con't.

Adenosine has an inhibitory effect on the **central nervous system (CNS)**, and endogenous adenosine also helps **cartilage** and inhibits the progression of osteoarthritis **("Endogenous Adenosine Maintains Cartilage Homeostasis and Endogenous Adenosine Inhibits Osteoarthritis Progression", *Nature*, Feb. 21, 2017).**

http://www.nature.com/articles/ncomms15019

Acupuncture Affects Blood Flow

In Traditional Chinese Medicine, the **health** of a person **depends** on the ability to **generate nutrient-dense, oxygenated blood** and **move** this **blood** to every part of the **body**. In fact, **aging** is considered a **degradation** of the **vascular system** and its ability to create and transport healthy blood to all of the tissues. This makes perfect sense, especially when you look at all the roles of the human vascular system.

Table 1: Roles of the Vascular System
("Vascular Model of Disease Pathogenesis", *Medical Acupuncture*, V27, No.2, April 2015)

Cancer Surveillance System	Endocrine System
Immune System	Coagulation System
Microvascular Perfusion Pressure	Neurotransmitters
Neuromodulators	Regulation of Cellular Metabolome
Regulation of Blood Pressure	Regulation of Body pH
Removal of Cellular Waste	Systemic Blood Pressure
Tissue Oxygenation	Tissue Nourishment

Studies show acupuncture can increase blood circulation **("Evaluation of the Effects of Acupuncture on Blood Flow in Humans with Ultrasound Color Doppler Imaging", *Evid Based Alternat Med.* 2012; 2012:513638).**
https://www.ncbi.nlm.nih.gov/pmc/articles/PMC3388479/

Further, acupuncture has been shown to improve the ability of heart failure patients to exercise and recover from exercise **(Acupuncture Improves Exercise Tolerance of Patients with Heart Failure: A Placebo-Controlled Pilot Study", *Heart*, 2010 Sep; 96(17):1396-400).**
https://www.sciencedaily.com/releases/2010/07/100701103409.htm

Dive Deeper into Biomedicine- Acupuncture as Anti-Aging Medicine

According to Traditional Chinese Medicine, **aging** is thought of as the **degeneration** of the **cardiovascular system,** and a key to **longevity** is to preserve and maintain the **manufacture** and **circulation** of **highly nutritious, oxygenated blood.**

Modern medical doctors would agree. In fact, **Dr. Edward Neal** states "**Impairments** in blood circulation represent a "**common pathway**" in **disease pathogenesis.** Disruptions of vascular circulation represent a functional "**gate**" through which all pathologic processes pass before they become a recognized illness. This suggests that previously diverse and unrelated categories of human illness can potentially be treated by a single and unified therapeutic protocol- **target regulation** of the body's **micro-** and **macrovascular circulations**" **(Vascular Model of Disease Pathogenesis, *Medical Acupuncture*, V27, No.2, April 2015).**

Acupuncture can promote many positive **hemodynamic** changes, including **cardiac output.** In a recent study, acupuncture stimulation at acupoint *Zusanli* (ST36) in healthy subjects "increased the peripheral pulse amplitudes (pressure pulse wave (PPW) and PPG), blood flow velocity (ultrasonography) and sympathetic nerve activity (HRV). The lack of changes in the AIX and PTT suggests that the increased pulse amplitudes and blood flow velocity may result from increased cardiac output" **("Hemodynamic Changes Caused by Acupuncture in Healthy Volunteers: A Prospective, Single-Arm Exploratory Study", *BMC Complement Altern Med* 2017; 17:274). https://www.ncbi.nlm.nih.gov/pmc/articles/PMC5440909/**

Acupuncture has also been shown to be able to modulate autonomic cardiovascular responses by enhancing parasympathetic function **("Short Term Effects of Acupuncture to SP3 on the Autonomic Blood Flow Control", *Neurol Res.* 2010 Feb; 32 Suppl 1:37-42). https://www.ncbi.nlm.nih.gov/pubmed/20034443**

Finally, acupuncture has even been shown to affect the blood flow in the brain **("Effects of Acupuncture on the Brain Hemodynamics", *Auton Neurosci*, 2010 Oct 28; 157(1-2): 74-80). https://www.ncbi.nlm.nih.gov/pubmed/20605114**

Acupuncture Affects the Central Nervous System (CNS)

Imaging technologies, such as **functional magnetic imaging (fMRI)** and **positron emission tomography (PET)** have made it possible to visualize cerebral activities and how acupuncture affects the brain.

Newer studies using this technology have helped show how acupuncture improves stimulus processing in the **Central Nervous System (CNS).** These amazing studies not only show that **chronic pain basically rewires the brain and over sensitizes the entire nervous system,** but also show that acupuncture can help to correct this **(Rewiring the Primary Somatosensory Cortex in Carpal Tunnel Syndrome with Acupuncture, *Brain*, 2017 April 1; 140(4): 914-927).** **https://www.ncbi.nlm.nih.gov/pubmed/28334999**

Dive Deeper into Biomedicine- Acupuncture Affects the Brain Via the CNS

Many other studies show that **acupuncture** affects **multiple regions** of the **brain**. This has helped to explain how acupuncture can affect the immune system, addiction, the endocrine system, and conditions such as nausea and vomiting, hypertension, obesity, Parkinson's disease, and diabetes, just to name a few. Examples include:

"Acupuncture on GB34 Activates the Precentral Gyrus and Prefrontal Cortex in Parkinson's Disease" ***BMC Complement Altern Med*** **2014 Sep 15; 14:336 https://www.ncbi.nlm.nih.gov/pubmed/25220656 ,**

"Acupuncture Modulates the Limbic System and Subcortical Gray Structures of the Human Brain: Evidence from fMRI Studies in Normal Subjects" ***Hum Brain Mapp*** **2000; 9(1):13-25 https://www.ncbi.nlm.nih.gov/pubmed/10643726**

"Acupuncture Modulates Temporal Neural Responses in Wide Brain Networks: Evidence from fMRI Study" ***Mol Pain*** **2010; 6:73 https://www.ncbi.nlm.nih.gov/pmc/articles/PMC2989943/**

Acupuncture Affects Molecular Biology and Gene Expression

Many **genes** in our body can be either turned on **(expressed)** or turned off **(inhibited)** by various factors in the **cells environment**. In fact, an entire new field of study called **"epigenetics"** refers to the study of biological mechanisms which can turn genes on and off. This means that just because someone is born with a specific gene, it does not mean they will have the trait that the gene is associated with. The gene either may or may not be expressed based on the environment that exists inside the body. In other words, a person may have inherited a particular DNA sequence, but specific genes in the sequence can be turned on and off based on the environment of the cells.

Both **acupuncture** and **electro-acupuncture** have been shown in to be able to affect the **expression** of certain **genes**. These studies show that is it entirely possibly to **"biohack**" your health using acupuncture.

Dive Deeper into Biomedicine- Acupuncture Genetic Biohacking

In a very interesting animal study, **asthmatic** rats were treated with acupuncture, and then their genes were analyzed for changes. The researchers concluded: "Our **serial analysis of gene expression (SAGE)** indicates that the gene expression profile of the **early airway response (EAR)** phase of **asthma** could be effectively and specifically regulated by acupuncture, which suggests that the gene expression of immune response and steroid hormone may play an important role in this treatment" **("Use of Serial Analysis of Gene Expression to Reveal the Specific Regulation of Gene Expression Profile in Asthmatic Rats Treated by Acupuncture",** ***L Biomed Sci*** **2009 May 6; 16:46).**
https://www.ncbi.nlm.nih.gov/pubmed/19419550/

Dive Deeper into Biomedicine- Acupuncture Genetic Biohacking Con't.

In another amazing study, researchers analyzed the gene expression profile of **normal** rats before and after a course of acupuncture (the course consisted of 7 acupuncture treatments given in a two week period). After the analysis of the data, the researchers stated: "In contrast to target-specific and one-way adjustment chemical reagents (drugs), acupuncture **upregulates various organ systems** that are **hypo-functional,** or **downregulates hyper-functional** systems. **Acupuncture is considered a mechanical signaling process.** Our results show that the essential effects of acupuncture on normal rats include the **regulation** of macromolecular biosynthesis, transportation, and metabolism. **Acupuncture orchestrates the activity of an organism by regulating the expression of specific genes"** **("Effects of Acupuncture on the Gene Expression Profile of Lung Tissue from Normal Rats",** ***Mol Med Rep.*** **2012 August; 6(2): 345-60). https://www.ncbi.nlm.nih.gov/pubmed/22580820**

Acupuncture Affects the Immune System

The **immune system** is a network of cells, tissues, organs, and other biological structures that work together to protect the body. Researchers at **Rutgers University New Jersey Medical School** reported that electro-acupuncture on an acupoint traditionally used to "strengthen the constitution" activated two nerve tracts in mice that led to the production of a natural biochemical that reduced infection in the mice.

In the study, the mice were fed a toxic bacteria which is known to kill them. Half of the rats received "sham" (fake) electro-acupuncture, and the other half received true electro-acupuncture. All of the sham group rats died, whereas half of the rats in the true electro-acupuncture group survived.

This led to the discovery of previously unknown **neuroimmune pathways** and is considered a **breakthrough** in neuroimmunology **(Can Acupuncture Curb Killer Immune Reactions? *Scientific American Mind*, May 2014). https://www.scientificamerican.com/article/can-acupuncture-curb-killer-immune-reactions/** . This is yet another example of how acupuncture research led to unexpected breakthroughs in biomedicine.

In another study, **impaired immune functions** (chemotaxis, phagocytosis, lymphoproliferation, and NK activity) in anxious women were significantly improved by acupuncture. Acupuncture brought their blood values closer to those of healthy people, exerting a modulatory effect on the immune system. **This same study showed that the most favorable effects of acupuncture on the immune functions appear 72 hours after the acupuncture session and persist for one month after the end of the complete course of treatment**.

("Effect of Acupuncture Treatment on the Immune Function Impairment Found in Anxious Women", *Am J Chin Med* 2007; 35(1):35-51) https://www.ncbi.nlm.nih.gov/pubmed/17265549

Dive Deeper into Biomedicine-Acupuncture Signals Neural Circuits to Regulate Immune System

Multiple studies have demonstrated that **neural circuits** are able to **modulate immune responses** by detecting inflammatory mediators and relaying signals back to the immune system. These studies results suggest a new anti-inflammatory mechanism exists, is mediated by the **sciatic** and **vagus nerves**, and modulates the production of **catecholamines** in the adrenal glands.

These studies also show that **electro-acupuncture** at the **sciatic nerve** controls systemic inflammation by inducing **vagal activation** which leads to the production of **dopamine** (dopamine has an **anti-inflammatory** effect in the **brain**):

"Regulating Innate Immunity with Dopamine and Electro-Acupuncture", ***Nature Medicine*** **2014 20, 239-241**
http://www.nature.com/nm/journal/v20/n3/full/nm.3501.html?foxtrotcallback=true

"Dopamine Mediates Vagal Modulation of the Immune System by Electro-Acupuncture", ***Nature Medicine*** **2014 20 291-295**
http://www.nature.com/nm/journal/v20/n3/full/nm.3479.html

Acupuncture Affects Neuromuscular Conditions

Neuromuscular Diseases are diseases which affect the **muscles** and/or their direct **nervous system** control. Problems with the central nervous system control can cause problems with **spasticity** or **paralysis**. Examples include Parkinson's disease, multiple sclerosis, and stroke. As previously stated, **acupuncture** can improve **signal processing** in the **central nervous system** and it has been shown to have a beneficial effect on neuromuscular conditions.

Examples of acupunctures effect on neuromuscular conditions include:

Animal study shows that electro-acupuncture produces **sustained motor improvement** for at least **four weeks** after treatment in mice with Parkinson's disease **("Electro-Acupuncture Produces the Sustained Motor Improvement in 6-Hydroxydopamine-Lesioned Mice", *PLos One* 2016 Feb 19; 11(2): e0149111). https://www.ncbi.nlm.nih.gov/pubmed/26894437**

Acupuncture can **reduce** the therapeutic L-dopa treatment dose and its related **side effect,** L-dopa induced **dyskinesia**, in patients with Parkinson's disease **("Acupuncture for Parkinson's Disease: A Review of Clinical, Animal and Functional Magnetic Resonance Imaging Studies", *Journal of Traditional Chinese Medicine,* V36, Issue 6, Dec 2015, pp709-717). http://www.sciencedirect.com/science/article/pii/S0254627215301643**

Acupuncture improved the time to walk 25 feet in patients with multiple sclerosis **("Effects of Acupuncture on Gait of Patients with Multiple Sclerosis", *J Altern Complement Med* 2017 Apr 14). https://www.ncbi.nlm.nih.gov/pubmed/28410453**

Acupuncture can improve **neuroplasticity** (the ability of the brain to rewire itself) in response to a stroke **("Enhanced Functional Connectivity between the Bilateral Primary Motor Cortices after Acupuncture at Yanglingquan (GB34) in Right-Hemispheric Subcortical Stroke Patients: A Resting-State fMRI Study", *Front Hum Neurosci* 2017 Apr 10; 11:178). https://www.ncbi.nlm.nih.gov/pubmed/28443010**

Acupuncture Affects Inflammation

The **anti-inflammatory** effects of acupuncture have been studied in in many inflammatory diseases including asthma, rhinitis, inflammatory bowel disease, rheumatoid arthritis, epicondylitis, complex regional pain syndrome, and vasculitis **("Anti-Inflammatory Actions of Acupuncture", *Mediators Inflamm* 2003 Apr;12(2):59-69). https://www.ncbi.nlm.nih.gov/pmc/articles/PMC1781596/**

Adenosine is believed to be a powerful **anti-inflammatory** agent that is generated by the body. In fact, the powerful drug used to reduce inflammation, **methotrexate**, is thought to be such a strong anti-inflammatory drug due to its stimulation of **adenosine release** in the body.

As stated earlier, animal studies demonstrate that after 30 minutes of acupuncture, concentrations of **adenosine** in the blood had risen to a level **24 times** greater than its baseline levels **("The Secret Behind Acupuncture", *Science Illustrated*, July/August 2011)**.

Studies also show that **electro-acupuncture** at the sciatic nerve **controls systemic inflammation** by inducing vagal activation which leads to the production of **dopamine** (dopamine has an anti-inflammatory effect):

"Regulating Innate Immunity with Dopamine and Electro-Acupuncture", *Nature Medicine* 2014 20, 239-241 http://www.nature.com/nm/journal/v20/n3/full/nm.3501.html?foxtrotcallback=true

"Dopamine Mediates Vagal Modulation of the Immune System by Electro-Acupuncture", *Nature Medicine* 2014 20 291-295 http://www.nature.com/nm/journal/v20/n3/full/nm.3479.html

Dive Deeper into Biomedicine- "Surround the Dragon" to Release Endogenous Adenosine

Topical treatment of **adenosine** to **foot wounds** in **diabetes mellitus** has been shown in lab animals to drastically increase **tissue repair** and **reconstruction.** Topical administration of adenosine for use in wound-healing deficiencies in humans with diabetes mellitus is currently being researched.

A Traditional Chinese Medicine acupuncture technique, called **"Surround the Dragon",** has been used for 2,000 years to accelerate healing in open wounds and infections. In this technique, the healthy tissue around a wound is treated by placing acupuncture needles locally around the wound. It is believed to produce its' positive effects at least partly through the local release of endogenous **adenosine** in the local tissue.

Acupuncture Affects Neuroplasticity, Hemodynamics of the Brain

Many medical conditions alter the structure, function, or blood flow in the brain. For example, in a **hemorrhagic stroke**, a blood vessel in the brain leaks or ruptures depriving brain tissue of oxygen and nutrients.

In another example, **chronic pain** causes frequent, strong pain signals and this abnormal "**nerve traffic**" actually causes **changes** in the **brain**, causing the **cortex** to get "**imprinted**" with the **pain signal**. This causes the person to **experience pain** even after the original cause of the pain has been repaired, and it also **sensitizes** them to **pain** in general.

Acupuncture can play an **important role** in helping the **brain self-repair**. Many hi-tech studies using ECG's, EEG's, and near-infrared spectroscopy have shown changes in the brain due to acupuncture needle manipulation **("Effects of Acupuncture on the Brain Hemodynamics",** ***Auton Neurosci.*** **2010 Oct. 28; 157(1-2):74-80).**
https://www.ncbi.nlm.nih.gov/pubmed/20605114 .

Further, multiple studies have demonstrated that **acupuncture** can assist the **brain** in **"rewiring"** itself:

"Neuroplasticity in Carpal Tunnel Syndrome", ***Journal of Pain Management,*** **V4, Issue 3**
https://www.novapublishers.com/catalog/product_info.php?products_id=25951

"Acupuncture Improves Outcomes in Carpal Tunnel Syndrome in Part by Remapping the Brain", ***Science Newsline,*** **March 2, 2017**
http://www.sciencenewsline.com/news/2017030218040042.html

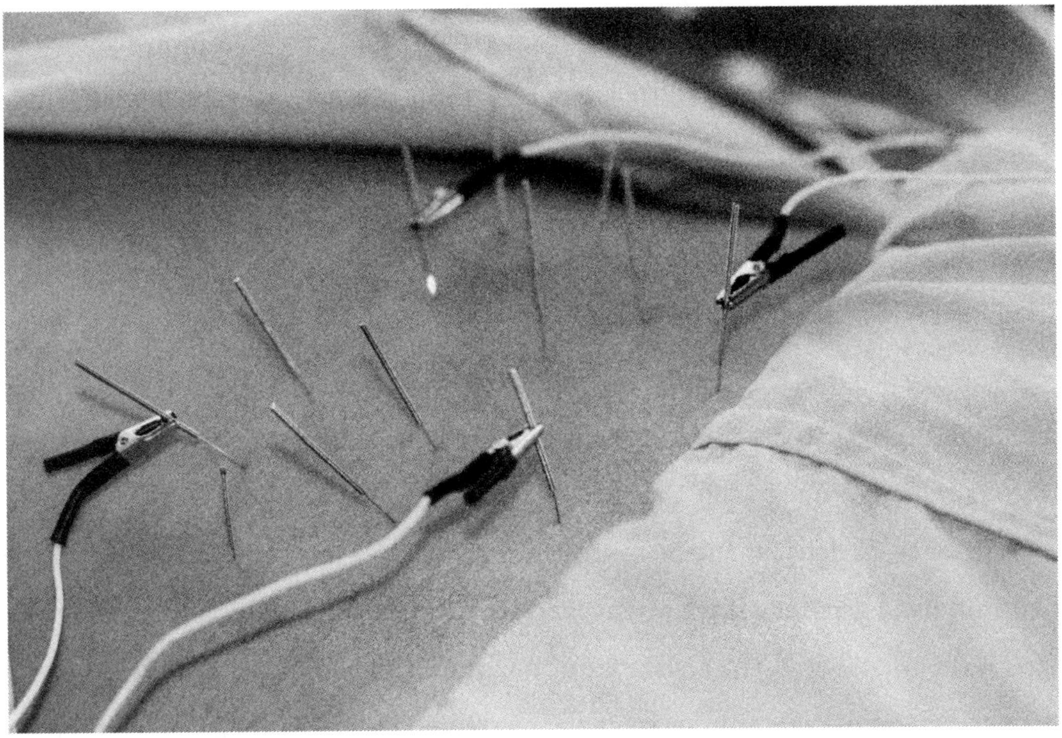

Electro-Acupuncture: Modern Advances In an Ancient Practice

Electricity has been used in healing since **2,750 BC** according to the oldest known stone carvings showing the use of electric fish for painful conditions in ancient Egypt. **"Electro-acupuncture"** is acupuncture with the addition of placing electrodes on the acupuncture needles and applying an electric current to the needles.

Modern electro-acupuncture was invented in China in the 1950's and was originally developed as a way for a doctor to treat more people in a shorter period of time. Instead of the doctor turning the needles by hand every few minutes, the machine can provide a constant stimulation, allowing the doctor to move on to the next patient.

Since then, the science of electro-acupuncture has grown significantly. It is now known that using **electro-acupuncture** at a **specific hertz** and **amplitude** can have very **specific effects** on **biological systems.**

Many people are familiar with **TENS** units and feel that electro-acupuncture is the same thing. But the two are **different** in several ways.

First, with **TENS,** a pad is placed on the **surface** on the skin and electrified. This does have clinical value, but the **electro-acupuncture** procedure has the added benefit of inserting a needle through the skin and getting the current **deeper** into the **tissue.** Skin has a natural electrical resistance, as does fat and bone. Muscles and nerves have less resistance, so the electric current has a **greater effect** when it travels through the acupuncture needle into the muscle tissue. In other words, the resistance of the subcutaneous tissues is low (because of surplus water), where the skin surface is highly resistant. Less **resistance** results in a **stronger biological effect**.

Second, different types of electric current are often used in electro-acupuncture, including **micro-current**. Micro-current is one millionth of an amp, and it is too low to incite nerve response (twitch) but it has **specific effects on a cellular level**. It is used for specific purposes, such as repairing a **connective tissue** tear. Placing micro-current on the skin does not allow the current to get deeply into the tendons and ligaments but electro-acupuncture gets the current exactly where it is needed.

There are other types of current used as well. **Milli-current** is what is used in a typical TENS unit and it is also used in electro-acupuncture. Instead of affecting cells, it has a broader effect on **muscles**, **tissue**, and **fascia**, but once again with electro-acupuncture the current gets deeper into the tissue. Milli-current is best to **strengthen muscle, improve local circulation,** and **reduce pain.**

Finally, **electro-acupuncture** combines the healing benefits of **acupuncture** with the healing benefits of **electrotherapeutics** to produce greater **clinical results** than either one alone.

Electro-Acupuncture Affects Molecular Biology and Gene Expression

Many **genes** in our body can be either turned on **(expressed)** or turned off **(inhibited)** by various factors in the **cells environment**. In fact, an entire new field of study called **"epigenetics"** refers to the study of **biological mechanisms** which can turn genes on and off. This means that just because someone is born with a specific gene, it does not mean they will have the trait that the gene is associated with. The gene either may or may not be expressed based on the environment that exists inside the body. In other words, a person may have inherited a particular DNA sequence, but specific genes in the sequence can be turned on and off based on the **environment** of the cells.

Both **acupuncture** and **electro-acupuncture** have been shown in to be able to effect the **expression** of certain **genes**. These studies show that is it entirely possibly to **"biohack"** your health using acupuncture.

Dive Deeper into Biomedicine- Biohacking Gene Expression with Electro-Acupuncture

Several animal studies have shown that **electro-acupuncture** at one specific point improved bone and made positive **biomechanical changes** by changing the **expression** of specific genes:

"Effect of Electro-Acupuncture on" *Mingmen"* (GV4) on Bone Morphogenetic Protein-2 Expression in Osteoporosis Rats" *Zhen Ci Yan Jiu* 2014 Apr; 39(2):130-5 https://www.ncbi.nlm.nih.gov/pubmed/24818497

"Electro-Acupuncture Stimulation at CV4 Prevents Ovariectomy-Induced Osteoporosis in Rats Via Wnt-B-Catenin Signaling" *Mol Med Rep* 2016 Mar; 13(3): 2485-91 https://www.ncbi.nlm.nih.gov/pubmed/26846191

Modulation of **gene expression** by **electro-acupuncture (EA)** was confirmed in an animal study that examined the effect of EA in rats with **hypercholesterolemia** (high cholesterol). In the EA treated rats, the effect of EA had the same effect on the **lipid profile** as Simvastatin (without the side effects!). The **global gene expression profile** showed that EA at an acupoint traditionally used for **fat loss** not only regulated the expression of genes that were responsible for **cholesterol metabolism** in the **liver** but also had an effect on expression of genes involved with signal transduction, transcription regulation, cell cycle, cell adhesion, immunity, and stress **("Modulation of Gene Expression in Cholesterol Lowering Effect of Electro-Acupuncture at *Fenglong* Acupoint (ST40): a cDNA Microarray Study", *Int J Mol Med,* 2007 Apr; 19(4): 617-629). https://www.ncbi.nlm.nih.gov/pubmed/17334637**

Electro-Acupuncture Releases Endogenous Stem Cells to Relieve Pain and Promote Tissue Repair

Stem cells are undifferentiated biological cells that can differentiate into **specialized cells** and can divide (through **mitosis**) to produce more stem cells. This means they are a special class of cells that can turn into any type of cell the body needs. For example, if you break a bone, stem cells can turn into new bone cells as part of the repair process.

Many **acupuncture** and **electro-acupuncture** studies have demonstrated that acupuncture and electro-acupuncture can promote the **production** and **circulation** of **stem cells** in the body. An overview of all the published medical literature regarding this was published in 2014. In the study, researchers concluded "Acupuncture results in beneficial effects in animal models of Alzheimer's disease, depression, spinal cord injury, and stroke, and that these effects may, at least in part, be associated with **progenitor cell proliferation** or **stem cell mobilization** in the **central nervous system (CNS)**. It is postulated that acupuncture/electro-acupuncture may have the potential to cause stem cell mobilization in humans" **("The Possible Role of Stem Cells in Acupuncture Treatment for Neurodegenerative Diseases: A Literature Review of Basic Studies", *Cell Transplantation*, V.23, pp.559-566, 2014).**
http://journals.sagepub.com/doi/pdf/10.3727/096368914X678463

Further, an amazing study published in the journal ***Stem Cells*** in 2017 showed that electro-acupuncture in rats, horses, and humans stimulated and mobilized **mesenchymal stem cells (MSC)** into **systemic circulation**. This resulted in **higher thresholds** for injury-induced pain and considerably increased a type of **collagen** that promotes **tendon repair** and **anti-inflammatory** cells known to be predictors of **faster healing time**.

As if that wasn't interesting enough, the same study showed that in **humans** the source of the stem cells was primarily **adipose tissue** (fat), while in **rodents** the tissue sources were more

heterogeneous, and that electro-acupuncture resulted in a **browning** of **white adipose tissue** in the rats.

It was also demonstrated that stimulating different acupuncture points caused very different effects (referred to as **"point specificity"**). Electro-acupuncture at immune acupuncture points in the **forelimbs** preferentially mobilized the **stem cells (MCS)** whereas electro-acupuncture at immune acupuncture points in the **hind limbs** mobilized **macrophages** (important cells of the immune system that are formed by a response to an infection or accumulating damage or dead cells) into the circulation **(*Stem Cell* 2017; 35: 1303-1315)**.
https://www.sciencedaily.com/releases/2017/03/170316174225.htm
http://onlinelibrary.wiley.com/doi/10.1002/stem.2613/full

Electro-Acupuncture Has Antioxidant Effects

An **antioxidant** is a molecule that **inhibits oxidation** of other molecules. **Oxidation** is a **chemical reaction** that can produce free radicals, leading to chain reactions that can **damage cells**. Antioxidants **terminate** these chain reactions.

Electro-acupuncture has been shown in a recent study to have an **antioxidant** effect and to help **protect** the **neurons** in the **brain**. Researchers in the study stated that because of this finding, electro-acupuncture is a **promising therapy** for Parkinson's disease **("The Antioxidative Effect of Electro-Acupuncture in a Mouse Model of Parkinson's Disease", *PLOS* May 23, 2011).**
http://journals.plos.org/plosone/article?id=10.1371/journal.pone.0019790

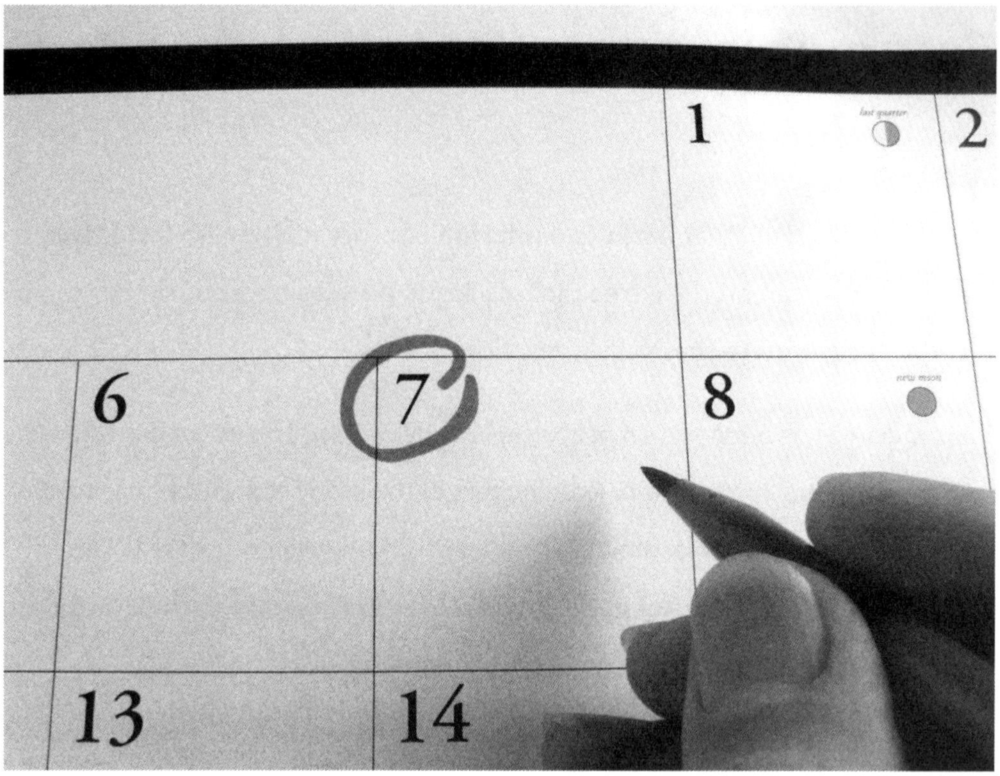

How Frequently Should I Get Acupuncture?

The **frequency** of acupuncture treatments **depends** on **many factors** including the condition(s) being treated, the severity of the condition, and how long the patient has had the condition, among others. But **generally** speaking, the **more acupuncture** a patient receives, the **better** the **outcome**. **Acupuncture is physical medicine.** In China, patients frequently receive acupuncture daily, and sometimes they even get acupuncture treatment twice per day. It's no surprise that outcomes of acupuncture in China are generally better than in America. It's not because the Chinese acupuncturists are better, it's because American patients typically don't get anywhere near the number of acupuncture treatments they actually need.

Subhuti Dharmananda, PhD, Director of the **Institute of Traditional Medicine,** addressed this issue in a proposal for restructuring American acupuncture practices.

Dr. Dharmananda states:

“Consider a few examples of other therapies. Is it appropriate to:

- Take a **nutritional supplement** (such as a vitamin/mineral/herbal formula) once per week, or once per day?
- Take a course of **antibiotic**s, one dose per week for ten weeks, or one dose per day for ten days?
- Take a **decongestant** once per week during allergy season, or every day during allergy season?
- Take an **antidepressant** once per week, or every day?
- **Exercise** 20-30 minutes once per week, or 20-30 minutes at least five days per week?
- Get a good nights **sleep** once per week, or every night?
- **Eat healthy** food once per week, or every day?

“At the beginning of a course of treatment, especially for a disorder that is severe or one that has been present for many years, it is very **unusual** (but not impossible) for a **single** treatment to trigger a **complete healing.** Instead, the treatment produces a **notable impact** (not always on the first treatment) that typically reverts after a day or two. This **reversion** is a result of the **continued presence** of **degenerative change**, **inflammation** (often systemic), **pathogens** (such as chronic viruses), **chronic stress, unhealthy habits,** chronic **poor nutrition**, **overwork**, etc. In other words, the **forces** acting to **counteract** the **therapeutic benefits** of **acupuncture remain active** long after the treatment effect wears off”.

“Further, **biochemicals** are released by acupuncture and have their effect, but they are **metabolized** and gone out of the system in a relatively **short** period of time. Acupuncture is like taking a complex drug of **neurotransmitters** and **immune response modifiers,** but taking the “drug” only once per week instead of daily is simply not enough” **(“Restructuring American Acupuncture Practices”, Subhuti Dharmananda, PhD, Director, Institute of Traditional Medicine). http://www.itmonline.org/arts/restructure.htm**

The single largest predictor of success with acupuncture is getting a high number of treatments over a short period of time.

A **good standard** for almost any condition is to complete one course of **ten treatments** within two to three weeks. **Complex disorders** typically require **more treatments** within a shorter period of time. But when patients get a lot of treatments within a short period of time, **amazing** things can happen.

For example, in one study acupuncture **every day** for **15 days** relieved diabetic peripheral neuropathy **("Fifteen Day Acupuncture Relieves Diabetic Peripheral Neuropathy", *Journal of Acupuncture and Meridian Studies,* June 2010, V3, Issue 2, pp.95-103). http://www.sciencedirect.com/science/article/pii/S2005290110600180**

In another study, patients with **bronchial asthma** were treated by acupuncture and had a **96% effective** rate. The frequency of their treatment was **30 treatments** over a three month period to initiate the effect, followed by **10 more sessions** per year to prevent relapse **("Anti-Inflammatory Actions of Acupuncture", *Mediators of Inflammation,* Apr 2003, 12(2): 59-69). https://www.ncbi.nlm.nih.gov/pmc/articles/PMC1781596/**

A study on the effects of **acupuncture** on the **immune system** of anxious women found that the **greatest effect** of the acupuncture **peaks** at **72 hours** after the treatment. It also found that the **positive effects** on the immune system lasted for **one month** after a course of **10 acupuncture treatments.** So in a case like this, it would be best to get acupuncture every three days for one month (10 treatments in a month), then take a month off and assess the results **("Effect of Acupuncture Treatment on the Immune Function Impairment Found in Anxious Women", *Am J Chin Med* 2007; 35(1):35-51). https://www.ncbi.nlm.nih.gov/pubmed/17265549**

Whenever acupuncture does not work, whether it's in a specific clinical case or in a published study, the first thing to look at is how frequently the acupuncture was administered.

There are times when you can get away with fewer treatments, such as when acupuncture is delivered as one aspect of a **treatment plan,** along with physical therapy, body work (such as massage therapy, myofascial release, etc), chiropractic care, yoga, nutritional support, herbal therapy, psychotherapy, and/or aggressive lifestyle change. **<u>But for those serious about recovery, more acupuncture is generally better.</u>**

Once I Finish a Course of Acupuncture Treatments, How Long Will My Results Last?

There are **many factors** involved in how long the results will last. For example, overuse injuries such as **lateral epicondylitis** (tennis elbow) may come back if the patient resumes the activity that originally caused the condition too soon. Other times the condition **never returns**.

But studies show that with **chronic pain,** the effects should persist after **12 months** as long as the patient is careful **("The Persistence of the Effects of Acupuncture after a Course of Treatment: a Meta-Analysis of Patients with Chronic Pain",** ***Pain*** **2017, V58, Issue 5, p. 784-793).**
http://journals.lww.com/pain/Abstract/2017/05000/The_persistence_of_the_effects_of_acupuncture.5.aspx

There are factors which influence the likelihood of the condition returning, and they are the same factors which influence the effectiveness of acupuncture in general (**see next section**).

Factors which Influence the Effectiveness of Acupuncture

The number one factor which influences the effectiveness of acupuncture is the frequency of acupuncture treatments (see "How Frequently Should I Get Acupuncture?").

Frequency of Treatment- The **number one factor** which influences the effectiveness of acupuncture is the patient receiving a **large number** of treatments over a relatively short period of time. Other factors which influence the effectiveness of acupuncture include:

Coffee, Tea, and Chocolate- **Methylxanthines** such as **caffeine** (found in coffee), **theophylline** (found in tea), and **theobromine** (found in chocolate) competitively antagonize **adenosine's** effects. As mentioned previously, adenosine is a powerful natural **anti-inflammatory** produced by the body. Acupuncture has been shown to greatly increase the amount of adenosine in the body. Because of caffeine's purine structure, it **binds** to some of the same **receptors** as adenosine. Therefore the effects of adenosine may be blunted in individuals taking large quantities of **methylxanthines** and the benefits of increased **adenosine** from acupuncture may be **reduced**.

Age – Generally speaking, **younger** patients **heal faster** than older ones, and they also have less **degenerative disease** as well. Further, there are specific acupuncture effects that are **reduced** with **aging,** such as **nitric oxide** (NO) production. This is important because nitric oxide plays a critical role in blood pressure, circulation, and other health processes. Acupuncture has been shown to increase the release of NO. Interestingly, gender and race do not influence NO release over the acupoints, but **age** and **obesity** do influence it **("Influence of Age, Gender,**

and Race on Nitric Oxide Release Over Acupuncture Points-Meridians", *Sci Rep* 2015; 5: 17547). https://www.ncbi.nlm.nih.gov/pmc/articles/PMC4664911/

Trycyclic Anti-Depressants- Research is showing that certain **pharmaceuticals** (specifically tricyclic antidepressants) can **positively** influence the effects of acupuncture for **some conditions** (typically pain). Research is currently being conducted to determine if other medications can enhance acupuncture's effects as well.

Self-Healing Potential of Patient- Some people generally heal faster than others. There are many reasons for this, including age, obesity, lifestyle, medications taken, chronic diseases (such as diabetes), and genetics. Those people that heal quickly are generally healthier and they also generally have better results with acupuncture.

Lifestyle- There are many lifestyle factors which influence the effectiveness of acupuncture, including activity level, fitness level, stress levels, diet, sleep patterns, alcohol abuse, smoking, etc. People who are fit, have a healthy diet, get regular sleep, avoid overwork, and avoid toxins such as cigarettes and alcohol generally have better results from acupuncture.

Obesity- Like age, **obesity** has been shown to **reduce** at least one action of acupuncture, which is the increase of **nitric oxide** (NO). This is important because nitric oxide plays a critical role in blood pressure, circulation, and other health processes. Interestingly, gender and race do not influence NO release over the acupoints, but **age** and **obesity** do influence it **("Influence of Age, Gender, and Race on Nitric Oxide Release Over Acupuncture Points-Meridians", *Sci Rep* 2015; 5: 17547). https://www.ncbi.nlm.nih.gov/pmc/articles/PMC4664911/**

Status of the Vascular System- In Traditional Chinese Medicine, the **health** of a person depends on the ability to **generate** nutrient-dense, oxygenated **blood** and **move** this blood to every part of the body. If the **circulatory** (vascular) system isn't healthy, the ability of getting nutrient rich, oxygenated blood to the tissues will be reduced. Acupuncture causes many **endogenous chemicals** to be released and these health enhancing chemicals are **carried** throughout the body by the **blood** in the circulatory system (See **"Acupuncture Affects Blood Flow"**). If the **vascular system** is damaged (by age, poor lifestyle, smoking, ect), the benefits of

acupuncture will be **reduced** and the number of treatments needed will go up. Luckily **acupuncture** can **improve** the **function** of the **vascular system** so every **treatment** will be **more effective** than the previous one.

"Healability" of the Condition- Some conditions are simply "**more healable**" than others. For example, while acupuncture can improve the symptoms of **multiple sclerosis** (MS), it will not "cure" it, regardless of how many treatments a patient receives.

Placebo and Nocebo Effects- The **placebo effect** is defined as when a person experiences an improvement in a condition due to their **expectations**, not from the treatment itself. The **placebo effect** is thought to be responsible for **50%** of the **positive results** of **prescription drugs ("Placebo Effect May Account for Half of Drugs Efficacy",** ***Live Science,*** **Jan 08, 2014). https://www.livescience.com/42430-placebo-effect-half-of-drug-efficacy.html**

There are many fascinating studies regarding this effect, and if fact entire books have been written on it and how to use it to improve your life (see **"You Are the Placebo" by Dr. Joe Dispenza)**. A short and simple (but interesting) **"Ted Ed"** video on the placebo effect for can be found here: https://www.youtube.com/watch?v=yfRVCaA5o18

The **"nocebo"** effect is when a person is conditioned to expect a **negative response** or to anticipate **negative effects** from an experience. One example is when a person experiences negative side effects from sugar pills, just because they thought they were taking a powerful drug. It is also when a person is convinced something will not work and therefore they experience that it didn't, even when objective data shows that it did. Some people simply do not want acupuncture to work, therefore it doesn't.

Both the placebo and nocebo effect can be extremely powerful. But the nocebo effect has been shown to be **even more powerful** than the placebo effect **("The Nocebo Effect",** ***SAAD Dig.*** **2016 Jan; 32:55-7) https://www.ncbi.nlm.nih.gov/pubmed/27145562** and has been used to explain the interesting phenomenon of **"voodoo death"** first discussed by **Dr. Walter Cannon** in 1942 **("Voodoo Death and Homeostasis: Brain-Body Unity Addressed"). http://www.medscape.com/viewarticle/750786#vp_3**

Dr. Cannon coined the term **"sympathetic storm"** to explain the negative effects of the mind on the body. This has wide ranging implications on how negative thinking can and does make people ill.

So the bottom line on placebo/nocebo effects is this: **All things being equal, patients who believe acupuncture will work generally have much better outcomes, while patients who believe acupuncture will not work generally have poorer outcomes.**

Part II:

What Conditions Can Acupuncture Improve?

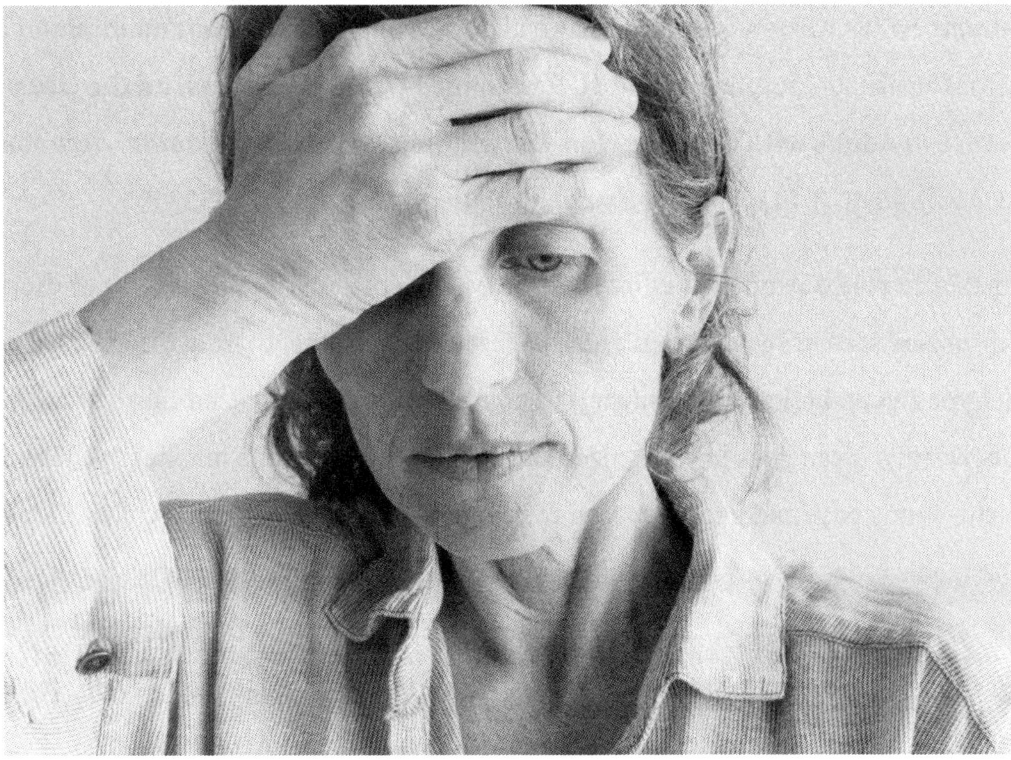

Anxiety

Anxiety disorders involve a state of distressing chronic but fluctuating nervousness that is inappropriately severe for the person's circumstances **(Merck Manual)**. Anxiety disorders affect over three million Americans each year.

According to **The Acupuncture Evidence Project**, acupuncture has "moderate" evidence supporting the effectiveness of treating anxiety. Acupuncture can be **safely combined** with conventional treatments such as medication or psycho-educational therapy, possibly **enhancing** their **beneficial effects** and **reducing** unwanted **side-effects**.

Acupuncture can often be effective for treating anxiety even in people who are "**non-responders**" to cognitive behavior therapy, bibliotherapy, and medication. In one study, non-responders were given one course of 10 acupuncture treatments. They showed significant

improvement on the Anxiety Inventory score and their improvement was **maintained** for **10 weeks** after the acupuncture treatments **("Randomised Controlled Trial on the Use of Acupuncture in Adults with Chronic, Non-Responding Anxiety Symptoms",** ***Acupunct Med*** **2015 Apr:33(2):98-101). https://www.ncbi.nlm.nih.gov/pubmed/25595195**

It is important to **rule out** other **medical causes** of anxiety (such as side effects of drugs, or medical disorders such as hypoglycemia, cardiovascular disorders, thyroid disorders, etc). For example, **hypoglycemia** (low blood sugar) is a common yet unrecognized cause of anxiety. In fact, hypoglycemia often goes unrecognized until extreme symptoms manifest. These patients go down the wrong path and get diagnosed for a mental disorder that is actually a blood glucose issue. The medications prescribed under these circumstances only lead to further complications. Here is a typical case report: **("Generalized Anxiety Disorder and Hypoglycemia Symptoms Improved with Diet Modification",** ***Case Rep Psychiatry*** **2016; 2016: 7165425). https://www.ncbi.nlm.nih.gov/pmc/articles/PMC4963565/**

Anxiety and **emotional disturbances** often lead to **immune system impairment.** In one study, **impaired immune function** in anxious women (chemotaxis, phagocytosis, lymphoproliferation, and NK activity) were **significantly improved** by acupuncture. Acupuncture brought their blood values closer to those of healthy people, exerting a **modulatory effect** on the immune system. This same study showed that the most favorable effects of acupuncture on the immune functions appear **72 hours** after the acupuncture session and **persist** for **one month** after the end of the complete course of treatment **("Effect of Acupuncture Treatment on the Immune Function Impairment Found in Anxious Women",** ***Am J Chin Med*** **2007; 35(1):35-51). https://www.ncbi.nlm.nih.gov/pubmed/17265549**

Acupuncture therapy for anxiety must be administered **conservatively,** especially at the beginning of a course of treatment because each patient has different **neural thresholds**, and if the needle stimulation is too strong, it has an inverse effect and increases anxiety **("Acupuncture for Treating Anxiety and Depression in Women: A Clinical Systematic Review",** ***Med Acupunct*** **2013 Jun; 25(3): 164-172). https://www.ncbi.nlm.nih.gov/pmc/articles/PMC3754836/pdf/nihms195439.pdf**

Dive Deeper into Biomedicine- Acupuncture and Anxiety

Research has shown that **acupuncture** treatment may specifically benefit **anxiety disorders** and symptoms of anxiety by:

Acting on areas of the brain known to **reduce sensitivity** to **pain** and **stress,** as well as **promoting relaxation** and **deactivating** the "**analytical**" brain, which is responsible for anxiety and worry **("Acupuncture for Treating Anxiety and Depression in Women: A Clinical Systematic Review",** ***Med Acupunct*** **2013 Jun; 25(3): 164-172). https://www.ncbi.nlm.nih.gov/pmc/articles/PMC3754836/pdf/nihms195439.pdf**

Regulating levels of **neurotransmitters** (or their modulators) and **hormones** such as serotonin, noradrenaline, norepinephrine, dopamine, GABA, neuropeptide Y and ATCH, hence altering the brain's mood chemistry to help combat negative affective states **("A Possible Mechanism Underlying the Effectiveness of Acupuncture in the Treatment of Drug Addiction",** ***Evid Based Alternat and Complement Med*** **2008;5(3):257-266). http://www.medscape.com/viewarticle/585219_3**

Stimulating production of **endogenous opioids** that affect the **autonomic nervous system.** Stress activates the sympathetic nervous system, while acupuncture can activate the opposing parasympathetic nervous system, which initiates the **relaxation response.**

Recommended Treatment Protocol: Physical exam and one course of treatment consisting of twelve treatments (3x/week for one month or 2x/week for 6 weeks). It is advised that the patient completes an Anxiety Inventory Assessment before and after the treatment to assess results. Additional courses of treatment may be necessary.

Treatment Goals: Rule out medical causes of anxiety, reduce intensity, frequency, and/or duration of anxiety as measured by Anxiety Inventory

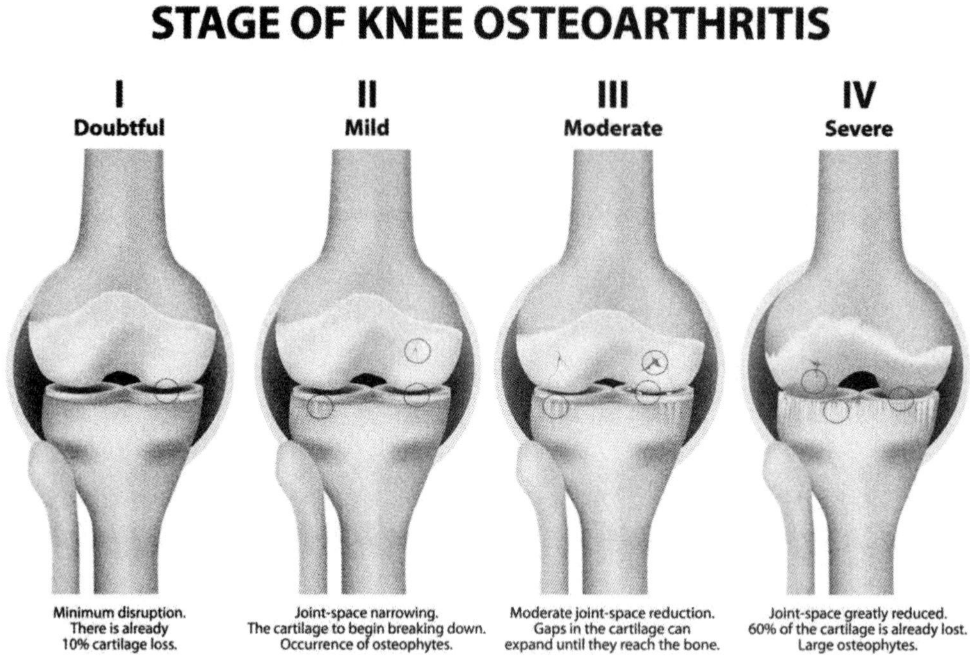

Arthritis

According to the **Arthritis Foundation,** arthritis is very common but not well understood. Actually "**arthritis**" is **not** a **single disease**, it is an informal way of referring to **joint pain** or **joint disease**. There are more than **100 different types** of arthritis and related conditions. People of all ages, sexes, and races can and do have arthritis, and it is the **leading cause** of **disability** in America. More than 50 million adults and 300,000 children have some type of arthritis. It is most common among women and occurs more frequently as people get older.

Common arthritis joint **symptoms** include swelling, pain, stiffness, and decreased range of motion. Symptoms may come and go. They can be mild, moderate, or severe. They may stay about the same for years, but may progress or get worse over time. Severe arthritis can result in chronic pain, inability to do daily activities, and make it difficult to walk or climb stairs. Arthritis can cause **permanent joint changes**. These changes may be visible, such as knobby finger joints, but often the damage can only be seen on x-ray. Some types of arthritis also affect the heart, eyes, lungs, kidneys, and skin as well as the joints. **(www.arthritis.org)**

Osteoarthritis (degenerative arthritis)-This is the most common type of arthritis. When the **cartilage** (the slick, cushioning surface on the ends of the bones) wears away, bone rubs against bone, causing pain, swelling, and stiffness. Over time, joints can lose strength and pain may become chronic. **Risk factors** include excess weight, family history, age, and previous injury (osteoarthritis typically starts at the site of a previous injury). **(www.arthritis.org)**

Chronically **tight muscles** apply physical pressure on joints which increases their rate of **degeneration.** Further, these tight muscles result in a **reduced blood supply** to the joints. Blood carries oxygen and nutrients to the joints, and low oxygen and poor nutrition reduce the natural ability of the joint to heal. One way **acupuncture** improves arthritis is by **relaxing** these chronically tight **muscles**.

When osteoarthritis affects a joint such as the knee, it results in subtle changes to the way a person walks and moves. This can cause further problems, such as low back pain and/or hip pain, and also increase the rate of **degeneration**, because of increased wear and tear on a joint that is moving in a way it wasn't designed to move. Acupuncture has been shown to improve gait in patients with osteoarthritis **("Immediate Effects of Acupuncture Treatment on Intra- and Inter-Limb Contributions to Body Support During Gait in patients with Bilateral Medial Knee Osteoarthritis", *Am J Chin Med*, 45, 23, 2017). http://www.worldscientific.com/doi/abs/10.1142/S0192415X17500033**

In multiple studies, **acupuncture** has also been found to be an **effective** treatment for **pain** and **physical dysfunction** associated with osteoarthritis of the knee **("Acupuncture and Osteoarthritis of the Knee: A Review of Randomized, Controlled Trials", *Fam Community Health,* 2008Jul-Sept;31(3):247-254) https://www.ncbi.nlm.nih.gov/pmc/articles/PMC2810544/ , ("The Effect of Acupuncture on the Symptoms of Knee Osteoarthritis- An Open Randomized Controlled Study", *Acupunct Med* 2004, Mar; 22(1):14-22). https://www.ncbi.nlm.nih.gov/pubmed/15077933**

Dive Deeper into Biomedicine- Acupuncture's Adenosine Increase Improves Arthritis

An interesting animal study demonstrated that **acupuncture** stimulates the release of endogenous **adenosine**, and that after **30 minutes** of acupuncture, concentrations of adenosine had risen to a level **24 times** greater than its baseline levels **(The Secret Behind Acupuncture, *Science Illustrated*, July/August 2011)**. Adenosine is widely found in nature and plays an important role in **biochemical processes**, such as **energy transfer**—as **adenosine triphosphate (ATP)** and **adenosine diphosphate (ADP)**—as well as in **signal transduction** as **cyclic adenosine monophosphate (cAMP).** It is also a **neuromodulator** believed to play a role in promoting sleep and suppressing arousal. Adenosine also plays a role in regulation of blood flow to various organs through **vasodilation**. Adenosine has an **inhibitory** effect on the **central nervous system (CNS)**, and endogenous adenosine also helps **cartilage** and inhibits the progression of osteoarthritis **("Endogenous Adenosine Maintains Cartilage Homeostasis and Endogenous Adenosine Inhibits Osteoarthritis Progression", *Nature*, Feb. 21, 2017).** **http://www.nature.com/articles/ncomms15019**

Inflammatory Arthritis (Rheumatoid, Psoriatic)- A healthy **immune system** is protective. It generates internal inflammation to get rid of infection and prevent disease. But the immune system can go awry, mistakenly attacking the joints with uncontrolled inflammation, potentially causing joint erosion and may damage internal organs, eyes, and other parts of the body. Researchers believe that a combination of **genetics** and **environmental factors** can trigger autoimmunity (smoking is an example of an environmental risk factor that can trigger rheumatoid arthritis in people with certain genes). **(www.arthritis.org)**

Acupuncture has an **immunomodulatory** effect. Researchers at **Rutgers University New Jersey Medical School** reported that electro-acupuncture on an acupoint traditionally used to strengthen the constitution activated two nerve tracts in mice that led to the production of a biochemical that reduced a **sepsis** (infection) in the mice. This led to the discovery of previously **unknown neuroimmune pathways** and is considered a breakthrough in neuroimmunology **(Can Acupuncture Curb Killer Immune Reactions? *Scientific American Mind,* May 2014).**

In another study, impaired **immune function** in anxious women (chemotaxis, phagocytosis, lymphoproliferation, and NK activity) were significantly improved by acupuncture. Acupuncture brought their blood values closer to those of healthy people, exerting a modulatory effect on the immune system.

This same study showed that the most favorable effects of acupuncture on the immune functions appear **72 hours** after the acupuncture session and persist for **one month** after the end of the complete course of treatment **("Effect of Acupuncture Treatment on the Immune Function Impairment Found in Anxious Women", *Am J Chin Med* 2007; 35(1):35-51). https://www.ncbi.nlm.nih.gov/pubmed/17265549**

Further, research has shown that acupuncture combined with a special herbal formula produces positive outcomes in RA patients **("Clinical Observation on Treating Rheumatoid Arthritis with the Guizhi Shaoyao Zhimu Decoction Plus Acupuncture", *Clinical Journal of Chinese Medicine,* 6.4 (2014):89-90). http://en.cnki.com.cn/Article_en/CJFDTotal-ZYLY201303013.htm**

Infectious Arthritis- A bacteria, virus, or fungi can enter the joint and trigger inflammation. Examples of organisms that can infect joints are **salmonella** and **shigella** (food poisoning or contamination), **chlamydia** and **gonorrhea** (sexually transmitted diseases), and **hepatitis C** (a blood-to-blood infection). In many cases, timely treatment with **antibiotics** may clear the joint infection, but sometimes the arthritis becomes chronic. **(www.arthritis.org)**

As mentioned above, acupuncture has an immunomodulatory effect. The **Rutgers** study **(Can Acupuncture Curb Killer Immune Reactions? *Scientific American Mind,* May 2014)** showed that electro-acupuncture helped mice fight off a deadly bacterial infection so it may be useful for infectious arthritis that has become chronic.

Metabolic Arthritis (Gout)-Uric acid is formed as the body breaks down **purines**, a substance found in human cells and in many foods. Some people have high levels of uric acid because they naturally produce more than is needed or the body can't get rid of the uric acid quickly enough. In some people, the **uric acid** builds up and forms **needle-like crystals** in the joint, resulting in sudden spikes of **extreme joint pain** (a gout attack). Gout can come and go in episodes or, if the uric acid levels aren't reduced, it can become chronic, causing ongoing pain and disability. **(www.arthritis.org)**

Gout's symptoms can be alleviated with acupuncture, but the best way to get rid of gout once and for all is through **metabolic treatment** and **diet**. Increased levels of uric acid are correlated with **high blood sugar** levels, so diet and lifestyle play large roles in gout. Also, **fructose** (including high fructose corn syrup), **alcohol** (especially beer), and **purines** (found is high concentrations in organ meats, beef, bacon, pork, and lamb) should be **avoided.**

Research shows that **tart cherry juice/cherries** are correlated with a **reduced risk** of gout attacks **("Cherry Consumption and the Risks of Recurrent Gout Attacks",** ***Arthritis Rheum*** **2012 Dec; 64(12):4004-4011). https://www.ncbi.nlm.nih.gov/pmc/articles/PMC3510330/**

While the evidence supporting acupuncture for arthritis is promising, more research is needed. Arthritis is a complex disorder requiring a large number of acupuncture treatments. As with any disorder, the number one predictor of success with acupuncture is a large number of treatments in a short period of time. Further, with all types of arthritis, it is best to start treatment early before the disease progresses. Unfortunately, as arthritis progresses, the usefulness of acupuncture will be reduced.

Recommended Treatment Protocol: Physical exam and one course of treatment consisting of twelve treatments (3x/week for one month or 2x/week for 6 weeks). Depending on the severity of the arthritis, additional courses of treatment may be necessary. **It is highly recommended that acupuncture is continually done on a regular basis ("maintenance") to slow the rate of degenerative change.**

Treatment Goals: Reduce intensity, frequency, and/or duration of symptoms associated with arthritis, and to slow further degenerative change and joint/tissue damage.

Pathology of Asthma

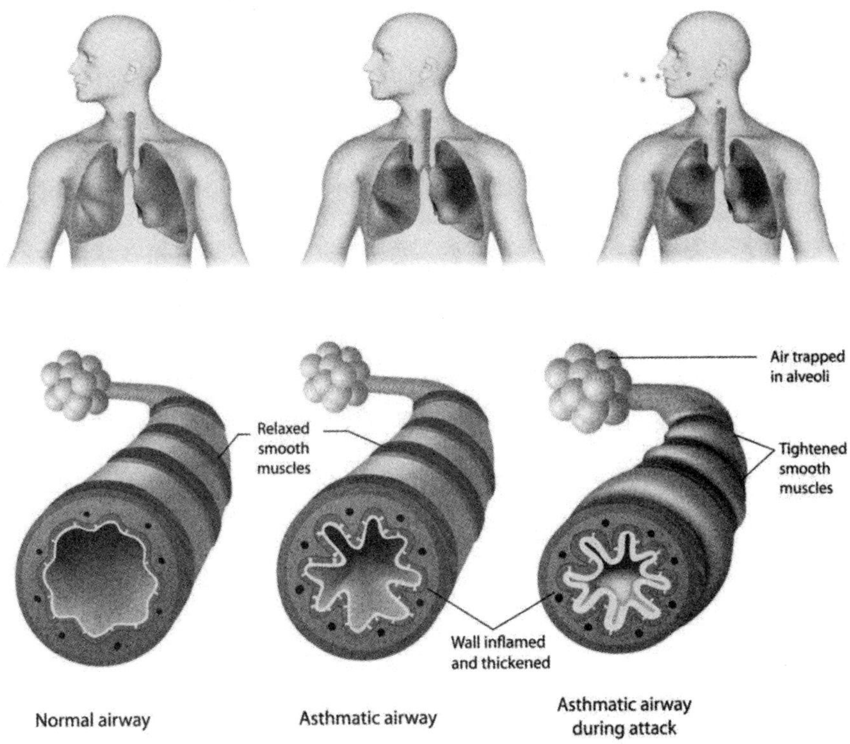

Asthma

Asthma is a common long term **inflammatory** disease of the airways of the lungs. It is characterized by variable and reoccurring symptoms, reversible **airflow obstruction**, and **bronchospasm.** Symptoms include episodes of wheezing, coughing, chest tightness and shortness of breath. These episodes may occur a few times a day or a few times a week. Depending on the person, they may become worse at night or with exercise.

According to **The Acupuncture Evidence Project**, there is "moderate" evidence to support the effectiveness of acupuncture to treat the symptoms of asthma in adults. Studies on the effectiveness of acupuncture for asthma have had mixed results, some extremely good and some showing very little effect. Remember, the number one factor which influences the success of acupuncture is a large number of treatments over a short period of time. Many studies in which acupuncture did not have good outcomes were studies in which the patients got too few treatments.

In one study, the use of acupuncture to suppress the daily intake of orally given corticosteroids and inhaled adrenergic agonists was investigated. This trial resulted in a good therapeutic effect **(96% effective rate)**. The investigators concluded that at least **30 sessions** in three months should be offered to initiate this effect, followed by **10 more sessions per year** to prevent a relapse. The extensive treatment with acupuncture in this study could explain the lack of effect seen in other studies **("Anti-Inflammatory Actions of Acupuncture",** ***Mediators of Inflammation,*** **Apr 2003 12(2); 59-69)**.
https://www.ncbi.nlm.nih.gov/pmc/articles/PMC1781596/

Dive Deeper into Biomedicine- Acupuncture Biohacks Asthma

Research has shown that part of acupunctures actions may be due to the effectiveness of acupuncture on regulation of **gene expression**. In a very interesting animal study, asthmatic rats were treated with acupuncture, and then their genes were analyzed for changes. The researchers concluded: "Our **serial analysis of gene expression (SAGE)** indicates that the gene expression profile of the **early airway response (EAR)** phase of **asthma** could be **effectively** and **specifically regulated** by **acupuncture**, which suggests that the gene expression of immune response and steroid hormone may play an important role in this treatment" **("Use of Serial Analysis of Gene Expression to Reveal the Specific Regulation of Gene Expression Profile in Asthmatic Rats Treated by Acupuncture",** ***L Biomed Sci*** **2009 May 6; 16:46).**
https://www.ncbi.nlm.nih.gov/pubmed/19419550/

Recommended Treatment Protocol: Physical exam and thirty (30) treatments over a three month period is considered once course of treatment. Following the initial three month period, treatments will be administered at least once per month to prevent relapse of symptoms. **It is advised that the patient be monitored by their primary care physician and/or their pulmonologist during the course of treatment**. Additional courses of treatment may be necessary.

Treatment Goals: Reduce intensity, frequency, and duration of the symptoms associated with asthma, reduce the amount of medication(s) necessary to maintain lung function.

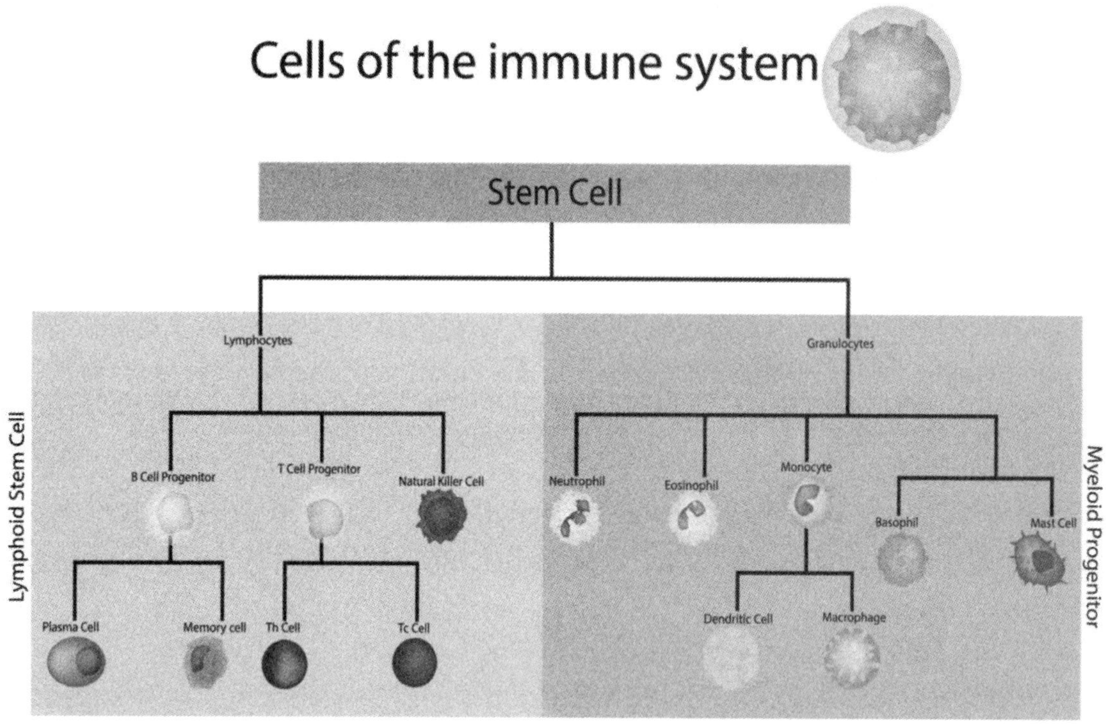

Autoimmune Disorders

The **immune system** is a network of cells, tissues, and organs that work together to defend the body against attacks by "foreign" invaders. Autoimmune disorders are disorders in which the body's immune system attacks healthy cells, treating as if they are "foreign" invaders. There are at least **80 types** of **autoimmune diseases**, including Rheumatoid Arthritis, Lupus, and Celiac Disease.

About 24 million people in the United States are affected by an autoimmune disorder, and women are more commonly affected than men. The cause of most autoimmune diseases is **unknown**. Treatment usually depends on the type and severity of the condition. **Nonsteroidal**

anti-inflammatory drugs (NSAIDS) and **immunoseppressants** are often used. While treatment usually improves symptoms, they do not typically cure the disease.

Research has shown that **acupuncture** can assist the body in **self-regulation** of the **immune system**. The results of a study on anxious women showed that the most favorable effects of acupuncture on the immune functions appear **72 hours** after the single session and persist **one month** after the end of the complete treatment.

The same study showed that impaired **immune functions** in anxious women (chemotaxis, phagocytosis, lymphoproliferation and NK activity) were **significantly improved** by acupuncture, and **augmented immune parameters** (superoxide anion levels and lymphoproliferation of the patient subgroup whose values had been too high) were significantly diminished. Acupuncture brought the above mentioned parameters to values closer to those of healthy controls, exerting a modulatory effect on the immune system.

Further, another thing that the study demonstrated is that **acupuncture facilitates** the **migration** of **cells** through the **endothelial layer** towards the infection **("Effect of Acupuncture Treatment on the Immune Function Impairment Found in Anxious Women", *Am J Chin Med* 2007; 35(1):35-51). https://www.ncbi.nlm.nih.gov/pubmed/17265549**

Modern acupuncture research has led to some major breakthroughs in **neuroimmunology**. Researchers at **Rutgers University Medical School** published a study which electro-acupuncture at a major acupuncture point (ST36) controlled a sepsis-related infection in mice. This study led directly to the discovery of one of the most intricate neuroimmune circuits found to date **(*Scientific America*, May 2014)**.

Dive Deeper into Biomedicine-Acupuncture Signals the Immune System Via Neural Circuits

Multiple studies have demonstrated that **neural circuits** are able to **modulate immune responses** by **detecting** inflammatory mediators and **relaying signals back** to the immune system. These studies results suggest a new **anti-inflammatory mechanism** exists, is mediated by the **sciatic** and **vagus** nerves, and modulates the production of **catecholamines** in the adrenal glands.

These studies also show that **electro-acupuncture** at the **sciatic nerve** controls systemic inflammation by inducing **vagal activation** which leads to the production of **dopamine** (dopamine has an anti-inflammatory effect in the brain):

"Regulating Innate Immunity with Dopamine and Electro-Acupuncture", ***Nature Medicine*** **2014 20, 239-241**
http://www.nature.com/nm/journal/v20/n3/full/nm.3501.html?foxtrotcallback=true

"Dopamine Mediates Vagal Modulation of the Immune System by Electro-Acupuncture", ***Nature Medicine*** **2014 20 291-295**
http://www.nature.com/nm/journal/v20/n3/full/nm.3479.html

Recommended Treatment Protocol: Physical exam and twelve treatments (2x/week for six weeks) is considered one course of treatment. Multiple courses of treatment may be necessary.

Treatment Goals: Reduce the frequency, intensity, and duration or symptoms associated with the autoimmune disorder.

The Facial Nerve

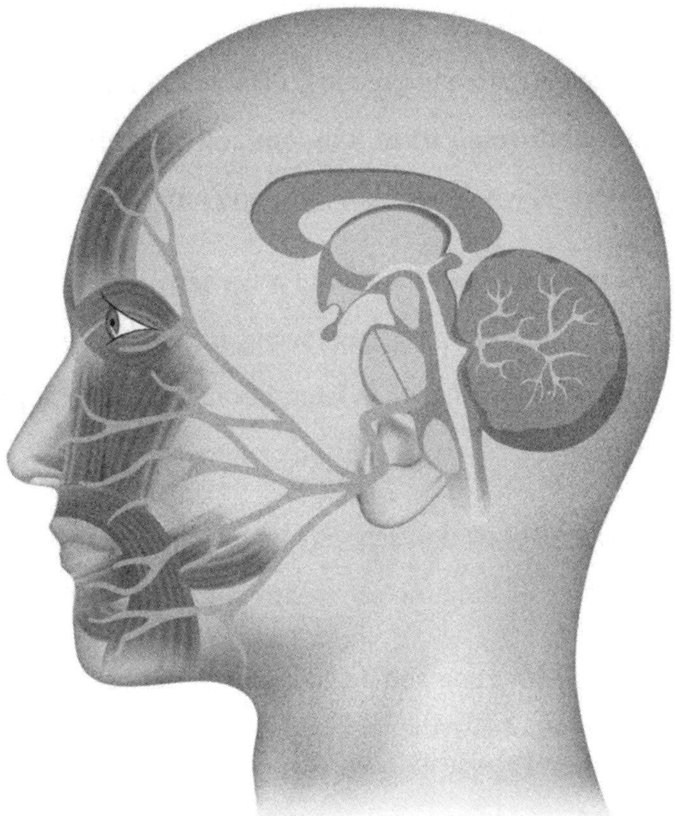

Bell's Palsy

Bell's Palsy is a neuropathy of the **facial nerve** (cranial nerve VII) and is characterized by weak or **paralyzed muscles** of **facial expression** on **one side** of the face. The cause of Bell's Palsy is unknown, but it is thought that it may be caused by a **viral infection** (even though anti-viral drugs haven't shown to be very effective in treating it).

Recent studies demonstrate that "**acupuncture** significantly improves **motor nerve conduction velocity** and **amplitude** and also promotes **functional nerve repair**" which may be one of the reasons acupuncture improves recovery from Bell's palsy **(*Neural Regeneration Research* V10, no. 1 (2015): 128).**
https://www.ncbi.nlm.nih.gov/pmc/articles/PMC4357096/

A review of all published medical literature regarding acupuncture for Bell's palsy was completed in 2015. After analyzing the data, researchers concluded "**Acupuncture** seems to be an **effective therapy** for Bell's palsy", but they also conclude that there are not enough high quality studies done and more research is needed **("Efficacy of Acupuncture for Bell's Palsy: A Systematic Review and Meta-Analysis of Randomized Controlled Trials", *PLos One*, 2015; 10(5):e0121880). https://www.ncbi.nlm.nih.gov/pmc/articles/PMC4431843/**

Acupuncture can **significantly shorten** the Bell's Palsy **recovery process**, reducing the suffering associated with speaking, chewing, swallowing, drinking, eye-closing, and sleeping. It is best to start acupuncture sooner rather than later, because the efficacy of acupuncture for this condition depends on the severity and duration of symptoms.

Recommended Treatment Protocol: Physical Exam and eight treatments (2x/week for 4 weeks) is considered one course of acupuncture treatment. Multiple courses may be necessary.

Treatment Goals: Reduce inflammation and begin repair of nerves, strengthen soft tissue, and improve local circulation to promote further healing.

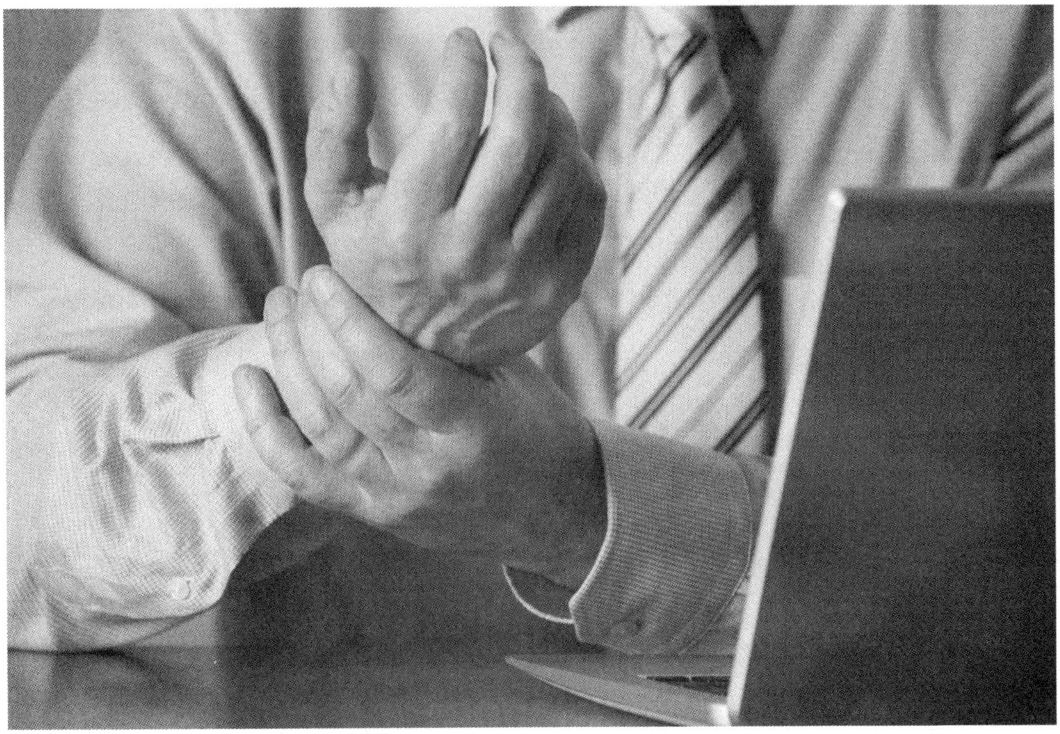

Carpal Tunnel Syndrome

Carpal tunnel syndrome (CTS) is a medical condition caused by **compression** of the **median nerve** as it travels through the wrist at the **carpal tunnel**. This leads to a range of **structural** and **functional changes**, which ultimately leads to **tissue damage** and **chronic pain**.

Risk factors include obesity, repetitive wrist work, pregnancy, rheumatoid arthritis, and possibly hypothyroidism and diabetes. It typically begins in adulthood and most patients are 40-60 years old. It is more common in women than men.

Permanent nerve, tendon, and muscle damage can occur if CTS is not treated. Early and proper **acupuncture** treatment of CTS not only relieves pain and numbness, it usually can **prevent permanent damage** to the wrist and hand. Since **other conditions** (carpal bone dislocations, rheumatoid thickening of the sheath, cervical radiculopathy) can mimic CTS, a physical exam is usually performed and in some cases a **nerve conduction study** will be completed.

Local acupuncture into the carpal tunnel itself helps to repair local tissue damage and reduces local inflammation, while **distal acupuncture** (needles inserted at specific acupuncture points away from the local site of injury) helps to improve **"neuroplasticity"** of the brain and helps the brain to undo the damage that strong pain signals, over a long period of time, can cause.

In other words, local acupuncture helps correct damage to the carpal tunnel itself (original cause of problem), while distal acupuncture helps correct the effects of long term pain on the brain by **"rewiring"** the brain (see **"Dive Deeper into Biomedicine- Acupuncture Rewires the Brain"**).

Dive Deeper into Biomedicine-Acupuncture Rewires the Brain

In any **chronic pain** situation, more **frequent** and **abnormal nerve traffic** to the **brain** results in **changes** in the brain in which the **cortex** gets "**imprinted**" with the **pain signal**. This results in the **experience** of **chronic pain**, regardless of whether or not the original source of the pain is still present. Further, there is a corresponding **hyper sensitivity** of the **peripheral nervous system**, making basically everything **hurt more** than it should.

There have been many studies involving how **acupuncture** can **reverse** this **process**, specifically in carpal tunnel syndrome:

"Neuroplasticity in Carpal Tunnel Syndrome", ***J Pain Manage*** **2011, 4(3):313-329**
https://www.researchgate.net/publication/287282522_Neuroplasticity_in_carpal_tunnel_syndrome

"Acupuncture-Evoked Response in Somatosensory and Prefrontal Cortices Predicts Immediate Pain Reduction in Carpal Tunnel Syndrome", ***Evidence-Based Complementary and Alternative Medicine,*** **2013**
https://dash.harvard.edu/bitstream/handle/1/11717680/3703406.pdf?sequence=1

Dive Deeper into Biomedicine-Acupuncture Rewires the Brain- Con't.

"Somatosensory Cortical Plasticity in Carpal Tunnel Syndrome Treated by Acupuncture", *Human Brain Mapping*, 2007 28:159-171) https://www.ncbi.nlm.nih.gov/pubmed/16761270

"Rewiring the Primary Somatosensory Cortex in Carpal Tunnel Syndrome with Acupuncture", *Brain*, V. 140, Issue 4, 1 April 2017, pages 914-927 https://academic.oup.com/brain/article-abstract/doi/10.1093/brain/awx015/3058778/Rewiring-the-primary-somatosensory-cortex-in

Recommended Treatment Protocol: Physical Exam and eight treatments (2x/week for 4 weeks) is considered one course of acupuncture treatment. Multiple courses may be necessary.

Treatment Goals: Reduce inflammation and begin repair of nerves, strengthen soft tissue, improve local circulation to promote further healing, and increase neuroplasticity of the brain.

Digestive Disorders- Lower GI: Irritable Bowel Syndrome (IBS), Ulcerative Colitis (UC)

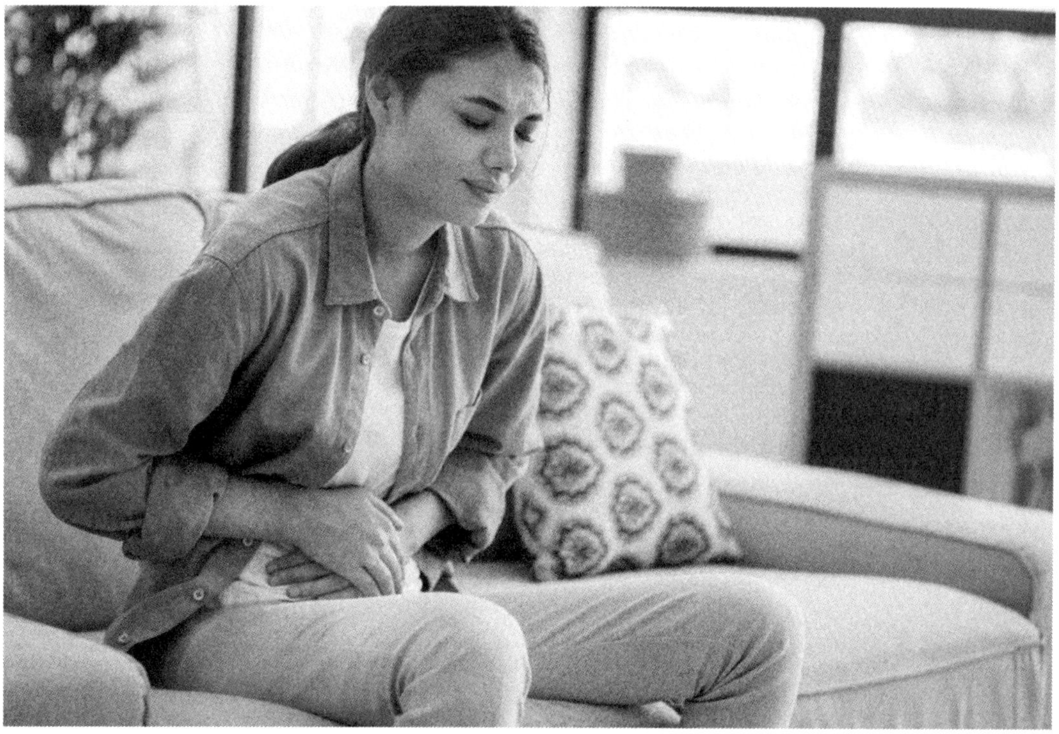

Irritable Bowel Syndrome (IBS)

According to the **Mayo Clinic**, **Irritable Bowel Syndrome (IBS)** is a common disorder that affects the **large intestine** (colon). IBS commonly causes cramping, abdominal pain, bloating, gas, diarrhea, and constipation. Even though signs and symptoms are uncomfortable, unlike inflammatory bowel diseases like ulcerative colitis or Crohn's disease, IBS doesn't cause changes in bowel tissue or increase your risk of colorectal cancer.

It's not known exactly what causes irritable bowel syndrome, but a variety of factors play a role. The walls of the intestines are lined with layers of muscle that contract and relax in a coordinated rhythm as they move food from your stomach through your intestinal tract to your rectum. If you have irritable bowel syndrome, the contractions may be stronger and last longer than normal, causing gas, bloating and diarrhea. Or the opposite may occur, with weak intestinal contractions slowing food passage and leading to hard, dry stools.

Abnormalities in your **gastrointestinal nervous system** also may play a role, causing you to experience greater than normal discomfort when your abdomen stretches from gas or stool. Poorly coordinated signals between the brain and the intestines can make your body overreact to the changes that normally occur in the digestive process. This overreaction can cause pain, diarrhea or constipation". **http://www.mayoclinic.org/diseases-conditions/irritable-bowel-syndrome/basics/definition/con-20024578**

With any digestive disorder, **trigger foods** should be **avoided**. Generally, patients with IBS can often benefit from a **gluten-free** and/or **low FODMAP** diet.

Acupuncture and **electro-acupuncture** can help with IBS. In fact, a recent study concluded "Electro-acupuncture is equivalent to loperamide (Imodium) for reducing stool frequency in IBS-D and FD patients" **("Electro-Acupuncture for Patients with Diarrhea-Dominant Irritable Bowel Syndrome or Functional Diarrhea", *Medicine (Baltimore)*, 2016 June; 95(24):e3884). https://www.ncbi.nlm.nih.gov/pmc/articles/PMC4998466/**

And according to a recent meta-analysis of acupuncture research, "acupuncture exhibits statistically and clinically significant control of IBS symptoms" **("Effectiveness of Acupuncture to Treat Irritable Bowel Syndrome: A Meta-Analysis", *World J Gastroenterol,* 2014 Feb 21;20(7):1871-1877). https://www.ncbi.nlm.nih.gov/pmc/articles/PMC3930986/**

Recommended Treatment Protocol: Physical Exam and sixteen (16) treatments, with ten treatments in the first two weeks followed by six treatments over the following two weeks. This is considered one course of acupuncture treatment. Multiple courses may be necessary. **Lifestyle modification (stress management, low FODMAP diet) may significantly reduce the number of treatments needed.**

Treatment Goals: Reduce the frequency, intensity, and/or duration of symptoms associated with IBS.

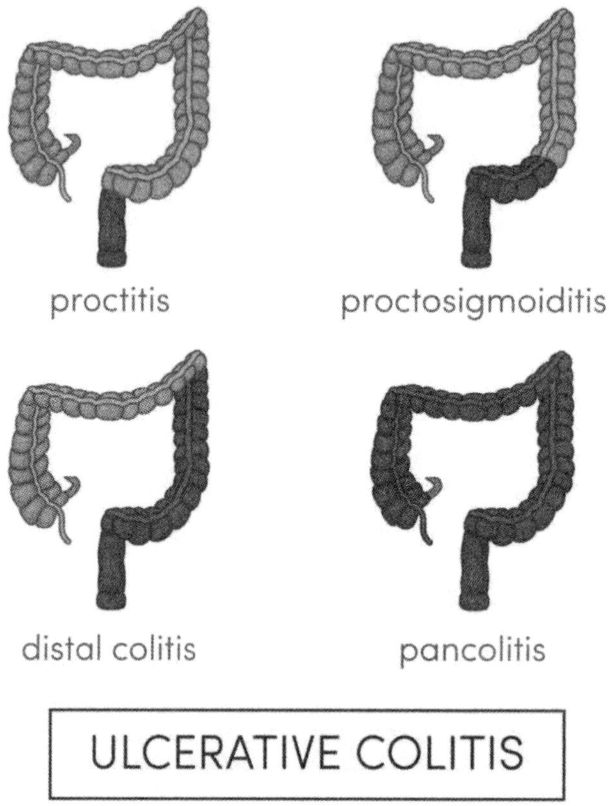

Ulcerative Colitis (UC)

Ulcerative colitis (UC) is an **inflammatory bowel disease** that causes long term **inflammation** and **ulcers** in the digestive tract. It affects the innermost lining of the **large intestine** (colon) and **rectum**. It can be **debilitating** and sometimes lead to **life threatening** complications. The exact cause of UC remains unknown, but one possible cause is a malfunction of the immune system **(Mayo Clinic)**.

Cytokines are substances that are secreted by certain cells of the immune system, and they have an effect on other cells. There are many types of cytokines. **Tumor necrosis factor-alpha (TNF-a)** is a cytokine that been shown to play a central role in the mucosal inflammation of the colon in both UC and Crohn's disease.

Electro-acupuncture has been shown to have a therapeutic effect on UC by reducing the concentration on TNF-a and alleviating inflammation damage **("Downregulation of Electro-Acupuncture at ST36 on TNF-a in Rats with Ulcerative Colitis", *World J Gastroenterol.* 2003 May 15; 9(5):1028-1033). https://www.ncbi.nlm.nih.gov/pmc/articles/PMC4611366/**

Recently, after reviewing all of the published medical studies, researchers stated "Clinical studies suggest that acupuncture and moxibustion therapy in ulcerative colitis (UC) can regulate bowel inflammation and these treatments have the advantages of low rates of adverse reactions and recurrence as well as long-term efficacy" **("Review of Clinical Studies of the Treatment of Ulcerative Colitis Using Acupuncture and Moxibustion", *Gastroenterol Res Pract* 2016; 2016:9248529). https://www.ncbi.nlm.nih.gov/pmc/articles/PMC5112307/**

Recommended Treatment Protocol: Physical Exam and 12 treatments (5x/week for 2 weeks, followed by 2x/week for one week) is considered one course of acupuncture treatment. Multiple courses may be necessary.

Treatment Goals: Reduce the frequency, intensity, and/or duration of the symptoms associated with UC, and to reduce and repair tissue damage caused by UC.

Digestive Disorders- Upper GI:

Low Gastric Motility (Gastroparesis), GERD

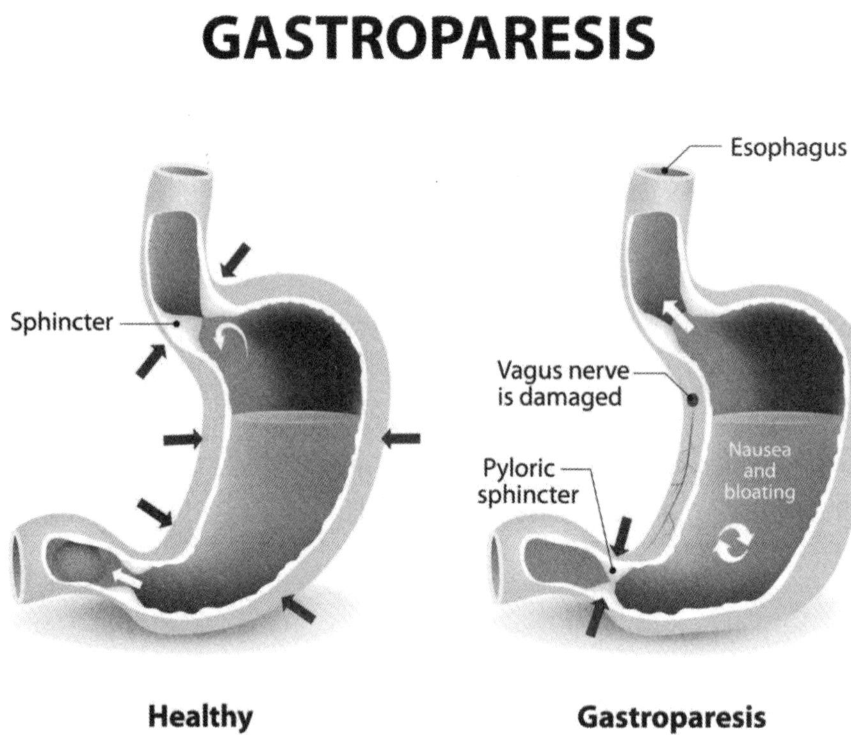

Low Gastric Motility/Gastroparesis

Low Gastric Motility, also called **gastroparesis**, is a condition that affects stomach muscles and prevents proper stomach emptying. In this condition, the nerves or muscles in the digestive tract do not function with their normal strength and coordination, resulting in a **reduced digestive function**.

Animal studies have shown that electro-acupuncture is **very effective** at regulating gastric motility **("Neural Mechanism of Gastric Motility Regulation by Electro-Acupuncture at**

RN12 and BL21: A Paraventricular Hypothalamic Nucleus-Dorsal Vagal Complex-Vagus Nerve-Gastric Channel Pathway", *World J Gastroenterol.* 2015 Dec 28; 21(48): 13480-13489). https://www.ncbi.nlm.nih.gov/pmc/articles/PMC4690177/

Recommended Treatment Protocol: Physical Exam and 12 treatments (5x/week for 2 weeks, followed by 2x/week for one week) is considered one course of acupuncture treatment. Multiple courses may be necessary.

Treatment Goals: Increase the gastric motility, reduce symptoms associated with gastroparesis.

Gastroesophageal Reflux Disease (GERD)

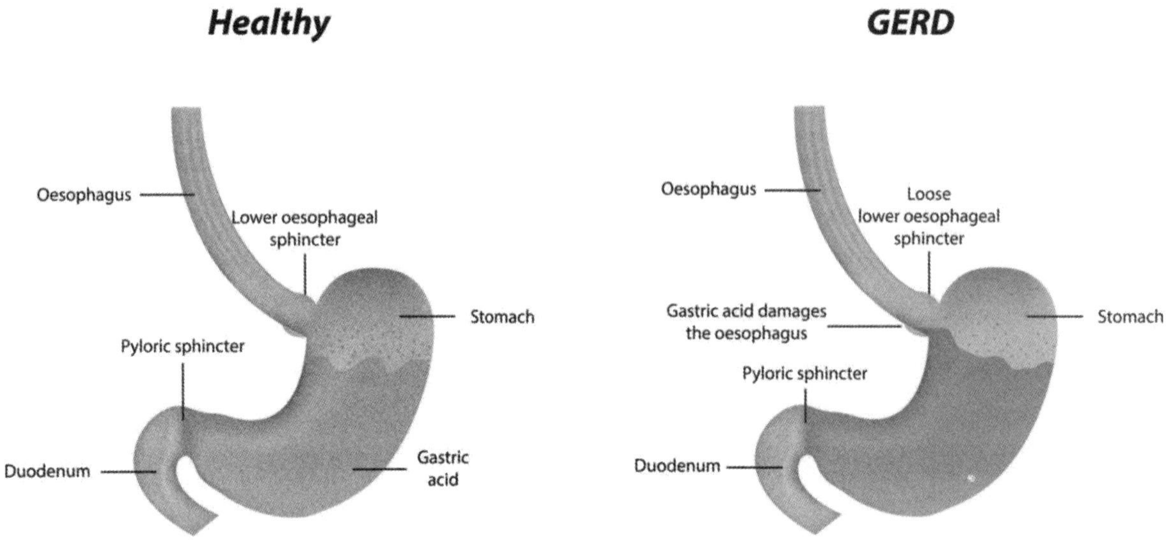

Gastroesophageal Reflux Disease (GERD)

Gastroesophageal reflux disease (GERD) is a **digestive disorder** that affects the lower **esophageal sphincter**. A problem with this sphincter results in **stomach acid** and **food** content **back flowing** into the esophagus. This backwash is very acidic, causing irritation to the lining of the esophagus.

According to a recent review of the published medical research, acupuncture has been shown to be effective and safe for the treatment of GERD **("Acupuncture for Treatment of Gastro-Esophageal Reflux Disease: A Systematic Review and Meta-Analysis",** ***BMJ*** **Original paper, Jul 7, 2016). http://aim.bmj.com/content/early/2017/07/07/acupmed-2016-011205.share**

Dive Deeper into Biomedicine-New Insights into GERD

New research is showing that contrary to popular belief, **low stomach acid** and **bacterial overgrowth** from a **high carbohydrate diet** are responsible for GERD:

"Improvement of Gastroesophageal Reflux Disease After Initiation of a Low Carbohydrate Diet: Five Brief Case Reports", *Altern Ther Health Med 2001* Nov-Dec; 7(6): 120, 116-9 https://www.ncbi.nlm.nih.gov/pubmed/11712463

"A Very-Low Carbohydrate Diet Improves Gastroesophageal Disease and it's Symptoms", *Digestive Diseases and Sciences*, V51, Issue 8, pp1307-1312 https://link.springer.com/article/10.1007%2Fs10620-005-9027-7?LI=true

Acupuncturist, author, and Functional Medicine expert **Chris Kresser** has excellent information on the relationship of carbohydrates, bacteria, and stomach acid which can be found here: **https://chriskresser.com/what-everybody-ought-to-know-but-doesnt-about-heartburn-gerd/**

Recommended Treatment Protocol: Physical Exam and 12 treatments (5x/week for 2 weeks, followed by 2x/week for one week) is considered one course of acupuncture treatment. Multiple courses may be necessary.

Treatment Goals: Reduce the frequency, intensity, and/or duration of the symptoms associated with GERD, and to reduce and repair tissue damage caused by GERD.

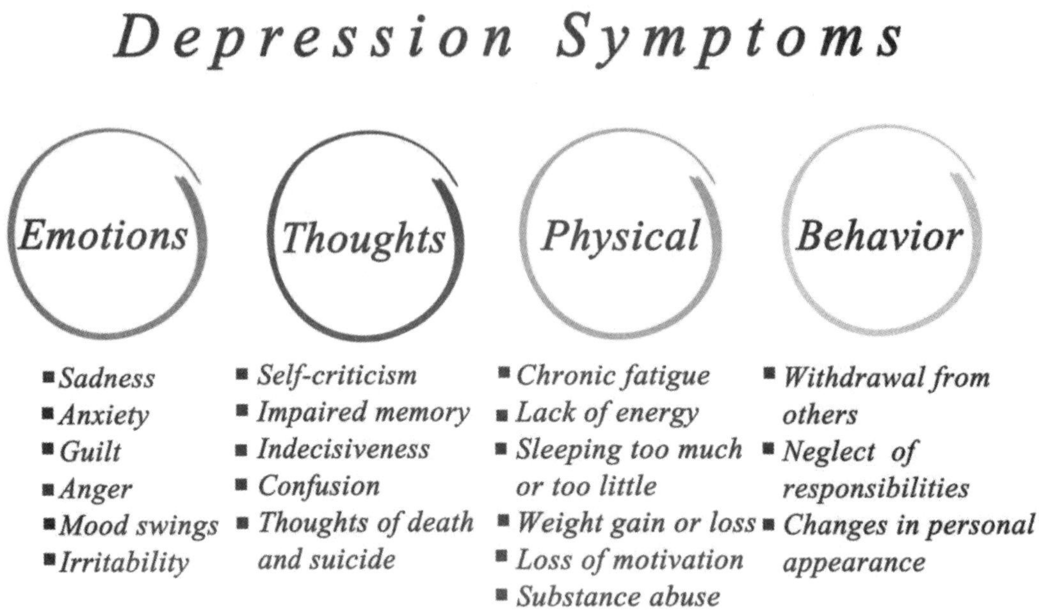

Depression

Depression is a **mood disorder** that causes a persistent feeling of **sadness** and **loss of interest**. It affects how you feel, think, and behave, and can lead to a variety of **emotional** and **physical** problems.

A number of **factors** may make a person more likely to experience depression, such as side effects of certain **drugs**, **heredit**y, **emotionally distressing events, nutritional disorders** (especially vitamin B6 and/or vitamin B12 deficiency), and certain **medical conditions** (hormonal disorders, infections, connective tissue diseases, neurological disorders, and some cancers). **A physical exam by a medical doctor is always recommended for people who feel they are depressed.**

It has been reported that **50%-60%** of patients with depression **do not respond to medication** completely. Moreover, because of the high incidence of **side effects,** many patients quit taking anti-depressant medication.

Recent systematic reviews of the published literature suggest that **acupuncture** increases **therapeutic efficacy** of **anti-depressants** and was proven to be a **safe add-on** treatment to depression. This is important because **less medication** equals less likelihood of **side effects** and therefore better **compliance** with medication **("The Benefit of Combined Acupuncture and Antidepressant Medication for Depression: A Systematic Review and Meta-Analysis",** ***J Affect Disord.*** **2015; 176:106-117). https://www.ncbi.nlm.nih.gov/pubmed/25704563**

Interestingly, a recent study compared **electro-acupuncture** to Prozac for reducing depression symptoms. Electro-acupuncture had a **faster onset of action, better response rate, and better improvement rate** than Prozac and with **no side effects**.

Further, in the same study electro-acupuncture also restored **GDNF** (a neuroprotective protein which is reduced in depressed patients) to **normal** levels **("Effects of Electro-Acupuncture on Depression and the Production of Glial Cell Line-Derived Neurotropic Factor Compared with Fluoxetine: A Randomized Controlled Pilot Study",** ***J Altern Complement Med*** **2013 Sep; 19(9) 733-9). https://www.ncbi.nlm.nih.gov/pubmed/23647408**

These patients were treated five times per week for six weeks, for a total of **30 treatments**. This illustrates the relationship between clinical success and the number of treatments needed (see **"How often should I get acupuncture?"** for more information on the importance of doing a large number of treatments over a relatively short period of time).

Dive Deeper into Biomedicine- New Theories of Depression

The cause of **depression** is unknown, but there is **evidence** supporting several **theories**:

The Monoamine Hypothesis of Depression- Monoamines play an important role in regulating mood and cognitive functions. The most popular theory for depression today is that depression occurs because of **depletion** of monoamines in the brain, especially **serotonin.** Animal studies have shown that electro-acupuncture can raise serotonin levels in the brain **("Change of Levels of Monoamine Neurotransmitters and Their Main Metabolites of Rat Brain after Electric Acupuncture Treatment", *Int J Neurosci* 1981; 15(3):147-149). https://www.ncbi.nlm.nih.gov/pubmed/6171540**

The Stress Hypothesis of Depression- One of the major **predisposing factors** for depression is **stress exposure**. According to this theory, alterations in the **hypothalamic-pituitary-adrenal (HPA) axis** contribute to depression, and restoration of the HPA axis is crucial for recovery. HPA overstimulation has been shown to produce excess **cortisol** (a stress hormone). Excessive cortisol is **neurotoxic** and can cross the blood-brain barrier, causing **brain damage,** especially in the area known as the **hippocampus.** Structural alterations of the hippocampus are one of the most consistent findings in major depression.

Studies have shown that **acupuncture** can **normalize HPA** abnormalities in rats, so the effects of acupuncture modulating the HPA axis may be why acupuncture has shown success in treating depression **("Effect of Acupuncture Stimulation of Different Acupoint Groups on Levels of Stress Hormones and Serum Brain-Derived Neurotropic Factor in Depression Rats", *Zhen Ci Yan Jiu*, 2015,; 40(6):444-448). https://www.ncbi.nlm.nih.gov/pubmed/26887204**

The Neurotropic Hypothesis of Depression- Neurotrophins are a subfamily of **neurotropic factors (NTFs)** that regulate many aspects of **neuronal development** and **functions**. They regulate the development, maintenance, and function of the **nervous system.** They are crucial for normal adult brain function, and impairment of NTFs has been implicated in **mood disorders**.

Dive Deeper into Biomedicine- New Theories of Depression Con't.

Several studies have shown that both acupuncture and electro-acupuncture can increase the levels of NTFs in the brain **("Long-Term, High-Frequency Electro-Acupuncture Stimulation Prevents Neuronal Degeneration and Up-Regulates BDNF and mRNA in the Substantia Nigra and Ventral Tegmental Area Following Medial Forebrain Bundle Axotomy", *Brain Res Mol Brain Res,* 2001; 108(1-2):51-59). http://www.sciencedirect.com/science/article/pii/S0169328X02005132**

The Neuroimmune Hypothesis of Depression- Alterations of the **immune system** have been observed in many cases of depression. In addition, depression is more frequently found in people with immune disorders. **Cytokines** are substances that are secreted by certain cells of the immune system, and they have an effect on other cells.

This theory states that depression is caused by the increased production of **pro-inflammatory** cytokines, resulting in **oxidative brain damage.** Electro-acupuncture has been shown to decrease levels of pro-inflammatory cytokines **("Imbalance Between Pro- and Anti-Inflammatory Cytokines, and Between Th1 anf Th2 Cytokines in Depressed Patients: The Effect of Electro-Acupuncture or Fluoxetine Treatment", *Pharmacopsychiatry,* 2009; 42(5):182-188). https://www.ncbi.nlm.nih.gov/pubmed/19724980**

These theories reflect the **complexity of depression.** Multiple pathways seem to be involved in the **mechanism of action** of **acupuncture,** and these **mechanisms** may **work together** to produce the **antidepressant effect** of acupuncture **("Acupuncture for Depression: The Mechanism Underlying Its Therapeutic Effect", *Med Acup,* V28, No. 6, 2016). http://online.liebertpub.com/doi/full/10.1089/acu.2016.1180**

Recommended Treatment Protocol: Physical Exam and twenty (20) treatments (5x/week for 4 weeks) is considered one course of treatment. Multiple courses may be necessary. **Lifestyle modification, nutritional therapy, and herbal supplements may reduce the number of treatments needed.**

Treatment Goals: Reduce the frequency, intensity, and/or duration of the symptoms associated with depression.

Human Eye Anatomy

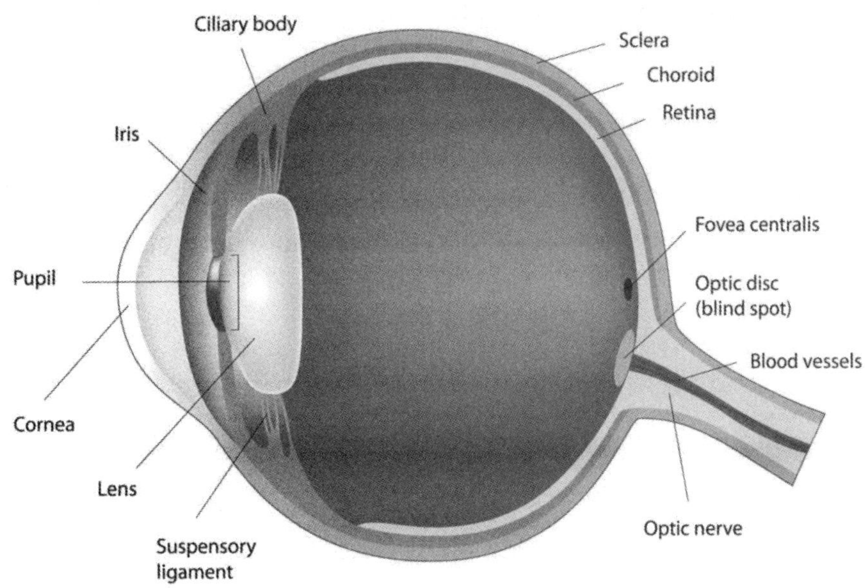

Eye Disorders

Eye disorders involve changes in vision, changes in the appearance of the eye, or changes in sensation in the eye. Eye symptoms typically develop because of a problem in the eye, but occasionally may indicate a problem elsewhere, particularly in the brain. **Eye conditions are frequently related to health conditions in the rest of the body.** In many cases, acupuncture can assist in improving and preserving vision. **For all serious eye conditions, it is important to be under the care of an ophthalmologist, optometrist, and/or medical eye specialist.**

Cataracts: A **cataract** is a clouding of the normally clear lens of the eye. Most patients with cataracts are told that there is **nothing** they can do so they ignore it until it gets to the point that they have to have **surgery**. But if cataracts are caught early enough, acupuncture, herbs, and supplements can slow and/or improve the condition.

Diabetic Retinopathy: **Diabetic retinopathy** occurs when **high blood sugar levels** cause **damage** to the blood vessels in the **retina.** It is a potentially blinding complication of diabetes, and in fact, it will affect approximately half of Americans diagnosed with diabetes. In this condition, it is very important to manage the high blood sugar levels in order to prevent further damage. However, with timely treatment, **90%** of even advanced diabetic retinopathy patients can be saved from going blind. Along with **lifestyle modification, medication, proper diet,** and **supplementation, acupuncture** can assist in helping those diagnosed with diabetic retinopathy.

Published case studies on diabetic retinopathy report "Results suggest that acupuncture plus herbal decoction had better therapeutic effect than western medications alone" **("Treatment of Diabetic Retinopathy with Acupuncture plus Herbal Decoction: Clinical Observation of 40 Cases",** ***Journal of Acupuncture and Tuina Science,*** **Dec 2004, V2, Issue 6, pp29-31).** **https://link.springer.com/article/10.1007/BF02848395**

Dry Eye: Acupuncture has been shown to improve symptoms of **dry eye**. In a recent study, acupuncture was given three times per week for four weeks (12 treatments). Acupuncture improved the symptoms of dry eye equal to artificial tears, but the acupuncture had the added benefit of increasing the **ocular surface disease index (OSDI)** and the improvements lasted at least until **8 weeks** after the treatments **("Acupuncture for the Treatment of Dry Eye: A Multicenter, Randomized, Controlled Trial with Active Comparison Intervention (Artificial Teardrops)",** ***PLoS One.*** **2012; 7(5): e36638).** **https://www.ncbi.nlm.nih.gov/pubmed/22615787**

Glaucoma: **Glaucoma** is a group of diseases that damage the eye's **optic nerve** (usually due to abnormally high pressure in the eye) and can result in vision loss and blindness. Ophthalmologist typically focus only on keeping the **intraocular pressure (IOP)** low, and this is important, but IOP is only one causative factor of progressive vision loss in optic nerve atrophy or damage.

Electro-acupuncture has been shown be very effective for **"normal-tension type"** glaucoma (manual acupuncture should only be used in patients with high IOP). In a recent animal study, researchers concluded "Electro-acupuncture provides **neuroprotection** by preserving retinal function in rats with experimental glaucoma" **("Electro-Acupuncture Provides a New Approach to Neuroprotection in Rats with Induced Glaucoma",** ***J Altern Complement Med.*** **2005 Apr. 11(2): 315-22). https://www.ncbi.nlm.nih.gov/pubmed/15865499**

In another study, manual acupuncture was used along with standard therapy on patients with **"open-angle"** glaucoma. After analyzing the data, researchers concluded "Acupuncture can improve the **retrobulbar circulation** and **intraocular pressure (IOP)**, which may indicate the efficacy of acupuncture for open-angle glaucoma" **("Short-Term Effects of Acupuncture on Open-Angle Glaucoma in Retrobulbar Circulation: Additional Therapy to Standard Medication",** ***Evidence-Based Complementary and Alternative Medicine,*** **V2011, Article ID 157090, 6 pages). https://www.hindawi.com/journals/ecam/2011/157090/**

Macular Degeneration: **Macular degeneration** (also known as **age related macular degeneration, or ARMD**) is the leading cause of **vision loss** in the U.S., affecting more than 10 million Americans. Macular degeneration causes vision loss in the center of the field of vision. In **dry** macular degeneration, the center of the retina deteriorates. In **wet** macular degeneration, leaky blood vessels grow under the retina.

Macular degeneration is one branch of a disease process that is based in **cardiovascular disease**. When dealing with ARMD, it is best to address the total health of the patient and lifestyle modification is a part of the treatment plan. Acupuncture has also been shown to have a beneficial effect in ARMD, and in one study it was shown to have an effective rate of over **88% ("Observation of Therapeutic Effect of Age-Related Macular Degeneration Treated with Acupuncture",** ***Zhongguo Zhen Jui.*** **2011 Jan; 31(1): 43-5). https://www.ncbi.nlm.nih.gov/pubmed/21355157**

Retinitis Pigmentosa: **Retinitis Pigmentosa (RP)** is a degenerative eye disease in which the **back wall of the eye** (retina) is damaged. It causes slow but progressive and permanent loss of vision. Currently, there is no medical cure for PR.

In an interesting study published in 2014, patients were given ten (10) standardized acupuncture treatments over a two week period. After the study, **50%** of the patients had measurable, significant **visual function improvement**. Researchers concluded "Acupuncture entails minimal risk, if administered by a well-trained acupuncturist and may have significant, measurable benefits on residual visual function in patients with retinitis pigmentosa" **("A Pilot Study of an Acupuncture Protocol to Improve Visual Function in Retinitis Pigmentosa Patients", *Clin Exp Optom.* 2014 May; 97(3): 240-247). https://www.ncbi.nlm.nih.gov/pmc/articles/PMC4018735/**

Recommended Treatment Protocol: Eye exam by a qualified medical provider and ten acupuncture treatments (5x/week for two weeks) is considered one course of treatment. Multiple courses of treatment may be necessary. **Maintenance treatments will be necessary in many cases.**

Treatment Goals: Recovery and/or preservation of visual function.

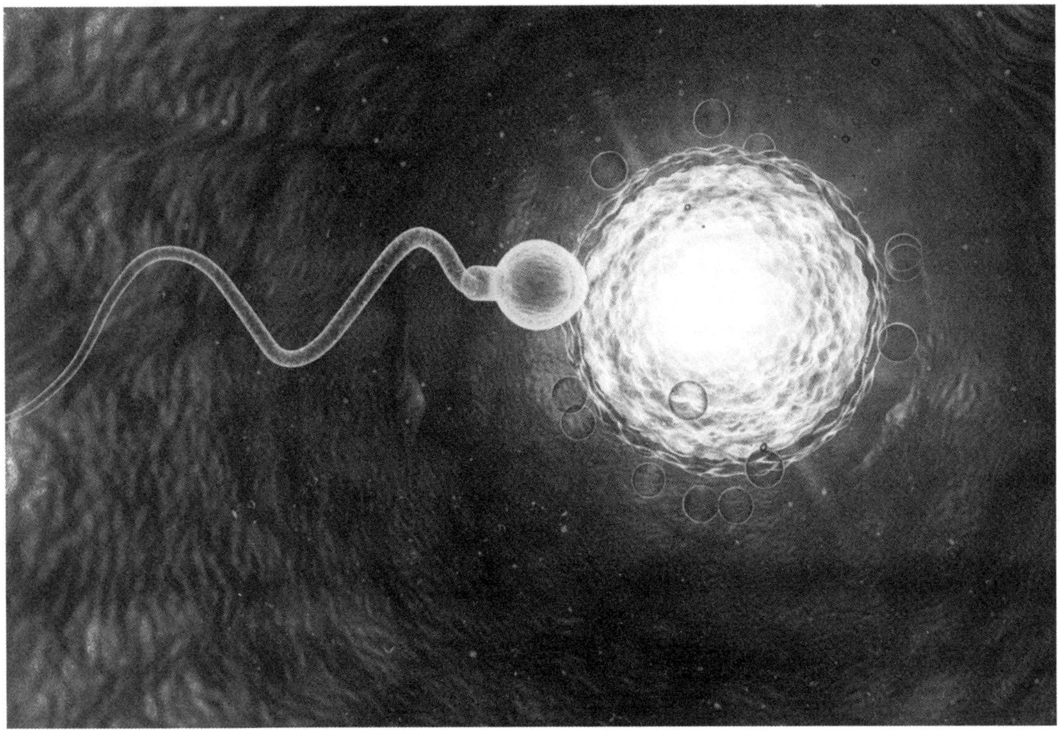

Fertility Support:

Female

Infertility is medically defined as the inability of a couple to achieve a pregnancy after repeated intercourse without contraceptives for one year. Infertility effects **one in five couples** in the U.S. and the **incidence is increasing**. Many factors have been identified including simple things such as people waiting longer to marry and have a child to much more complex things such as **hormonal disorders**, exposure to **drugs** and **environmental toxins,** and other **unknown** causes.

A review of the published medical studies regarding acupunctures effect on women's reproductive health was completed in 2014. After analyzing the data, researchers concluded "There is preliminary data indicating that acupuncture may improve menstrual health and

coping for women experiencing delays in falling pregnant. There is experimental data showing that acupuncture can influence female reproductive functioning, although the actual mechanisms involved are not yet clarified" **("Acupuncture and Women's Health: An Overview of the Role of Acupuncture and its Clinical Management in Women's Reproductive Health",** ***Int J Womens Health.*** **2014; 6:313-325).**
https://www.ncbi.nlm.nih.gov/pmc/articles/PMC3962314/

Researchers from **Weill Cornell Medical Center** in New York reviewed recent studies and concluded acupuncture specifically helps to:

- Increase blood flow to the uterus, which improves the chances of an ovum implanting on the uterine wall
- Reduce anxiety and stress. The hormones that are secreted during stressful situations can significantly decrease fertility
- Normalize hormone and endocrine systems that regulate ovulation, especially in women with PCOS
- Positively affect the hypothalamic-pituitary-ovarian axis, which plays a key role in fertility
- Regulate the menstrual cycle

Further, in 2008 the **British Medical Journal (BMJ)** published research which concluded that acupuncture can be offered as a significant, clinically relevant adjunct to **IVF**, relaxing the uterus and increasing blood flow for the successful implantation of an embryo within the uterine lining.

Dive Deeper into Biomedicine- Female Infertility Studies

PCOS: Acupuncture treatment resulted in higher ovulation frequency in lean/overweight women with PCOS **("Acupuncture for Ovulation Induction in Polycystic Ovarian Syndrome: A Randomized Controlled Trial",** ***Am J Physiol Endocrinol Metab,*** **2013 May 1; 304(9):E934-43). https://www.ncbi.nlm.nih.gov/pubmed/23482444/**

PCOS with IVF/ICSI: Acupuncture may increase the clinical pregnancy rate and the ongoing pregnancy rate and decrease the risk of **ovarian hyper-stimulation syndrome** in women with PCOS undergoing IVF or ICSI **("Effectiveness of Acupuncture in Women with Polycystic Ovarian Syndrome Undergoing In Vitro Fertilization or Intracytoplasmic Sperm Injection: A Systematic Review and Meta-Analysis",** ***Acupunct Med*** **2017 June; 35(3):162-170). https://www.ncbi.nlm.nih.gov/pubmed/28077366**

Endometriosis: Cochrane Reviews are systematic reviews of primary research in human health care and health policy, and are internationally recognized as the highest standard in evidence-based health care.

In a recent **Cochrane Review** of medical studies, researchers stated "The total effective rate of acupuncture for **endometriosis pain** was **91.9%** **("Acupuncture for Pain in Endometriosis",** ***Cochrane Database Syst Rev,*** **2011 Sept 7(9):CD007864). https://www.ncbi.nlm.nih.gov/pubmed/21901713**

All Infertility: The habit of **smoking** has been shown to **reduce** levels of vitamin B12 **("Relationship of Tobacco Smoking with Serum Vitamin B12, Folic Acid, and Hematological Indices in Healthy Adults",** ***Public Health Nutri.*** **2003 Oct; 6(7): 675-81). https://www.ncbi.nlm.nih.gov/pubmed/14552668**

Vitamin B12 is a water soluble vitamin that plays an important role in the functioning of the brain and nervous system. Symptoms of vitamin B12 deficiency are many, but can include a reduced ability to think, irritability, depression, inflammation, poor muscle function, and **decreased fertility**.

Recommended Treatment Protocol: Each clinical scenario is different, and the acupuncture protocol will be individualized to the exact medical presentation. **Generally speaking, fertility issues require at least three months of acupuncture treatment.**

Treatment Goals: Take home healthy baby.

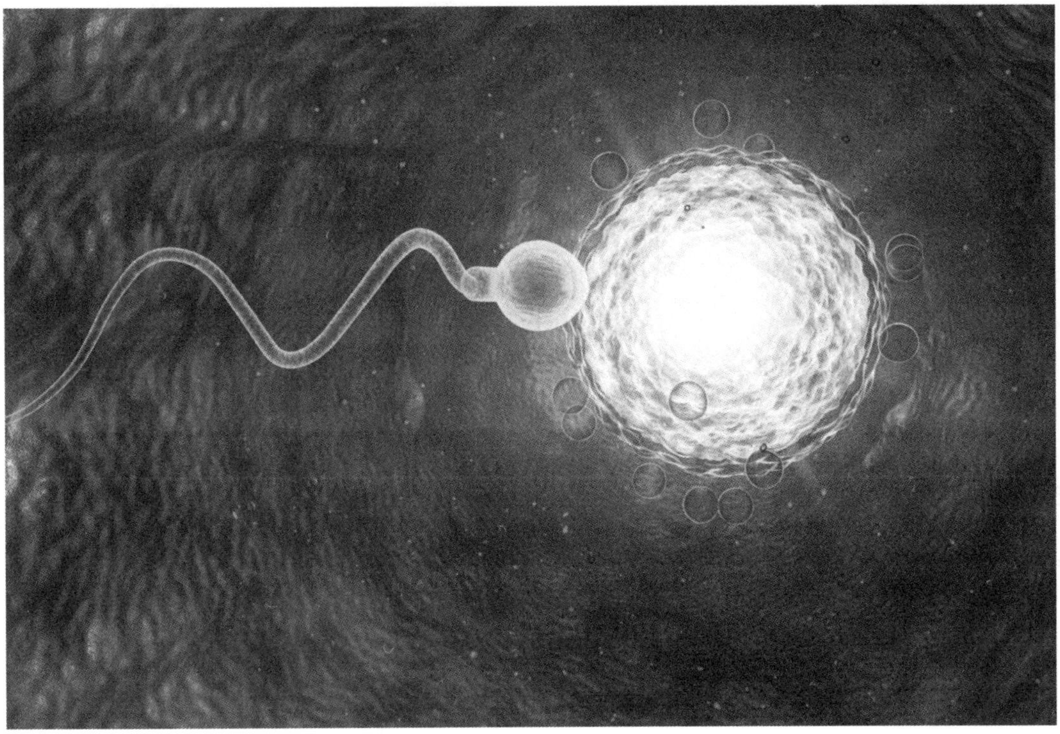

Fertility Support:

Male

Half of all couples struggling with infertility issues have a component of **male factor infertility**, and almost **30%** of infertility will be due **solely** to male factors. Male conditions that effect fertility are **under diagnosed and under treated,** and in **40%** of patients, **no medical cause** of male infertility can be found. Further, there are **limited medical options** available for treating male infertility, resulting in frustration for both medical providers and patients alike.

Acupuncture has been used in China for centuries to treat male infertility. The Emperors of ancient China desired enhanced virility and demanded the ability to produce many offspring, so royal acupuncturists developed very effective acupuncture treatments (and herbal therapies) as if their life depended on it. And in fact, it did.

Modern research is confirming what the ancient Chinese knew to be true. In one animal study, rats were first treated with heat to damage their sperm production, followed by ten sessions of electro-acupuncture. Researchers concluded there was a consistent trend of **improved motility,** and **increased number** of motile spermatozoa in the electro-acupuncture treated group compared to the control group. Also, electro-acupuncture **enhanced germ cell proliferation** through the improvement of **Sertoli cell** functions. They stated "Electro-acupuncture may facilitate the recovery of spermatogenesis and may restore normal semen parameters in subfertile patients" **("Electro-Acupuncture Enhances Spermatogenesis in Rats after Scrotal Heat Treatment", *Spermatogenesis* 2012 Jan 1; 2(1): 53-62). https://www.ncbi.nlm.nih.gov/pubmed/22553490**

In another study, acupuncture was given twice a week for five weeks (ten treatments total) to men with poor quality sperm. After ten acupuncture treatments, the semen from the men was analyzed and researchers concluded "A **general improvement** of **sperm quality**, specifically in the ultrastructure integrity of spermatozoa, was seen after acupuncture" **("Quantitative Evaluation of Spermatozoa Ultrastructure after Acupuncture Treatment for Idiopathic Male Infertility", *Fertil Steril* 2005 Jul; 84(1):141-7). https://www.ncbi.nlm.nih.gov/pubmed/16009169**

One thing that will improve the chances of a healthy conception is to **quit smoking.** The habit of smoking has been shown to reduce levels of vitamin B12 **("Relationship of Tobacco Smoking with Serum Vitamin B12, Folic Acid, and Hematological Indices in Healthy Adults", *Public Health Nutri.* 2003 Oct; 6(7): 675-81). https://www.ncbi.nlm.nih.gov/pubmed/14552668**

Vitamin B12 is a water soluble vitamin that plays an important role in the functioning of the brain and nervous system. Symptoms of vitamin B12 deficiency are many, but can include a reduced ability to think, irritability, depression, inflammation, poor muscle function, and **decreased fertility**.

Further, fathers who smoke **damage their DNA** and the effects are **passed down** to their children **("Cigarette Smoke Damages DNA in the Reproductive Cells of Fathers and these**

Changes are Inherited by the Offspring" (*Medical News Today*, June 26, 2012). https://www.medicalnewstoday.com/releases/246986.php

For more information on the importance of quitting smoking and how acupuncture can assist in this process, see **"Stop Smoking"**.

Dive Deeper into Biomedicine- Male Infertility Acupuncture Research Overview

A slightly dated (2005) yet still relevant discussion on the research on acupuncture and male fertility can be found here: **https://www.ahcmedia.com/articles/86519-acupuncture-for-the-treatment-of-male-infertility**

Recommended Treatment Protocol: Each clinical scenario is different, and the acupuncture protocol will be individualized to the exact medical presentation. **Generally speaking, fertility issues require at least three months of acupuncture treatment.**

Treatment Goals: Take home healthy baby.

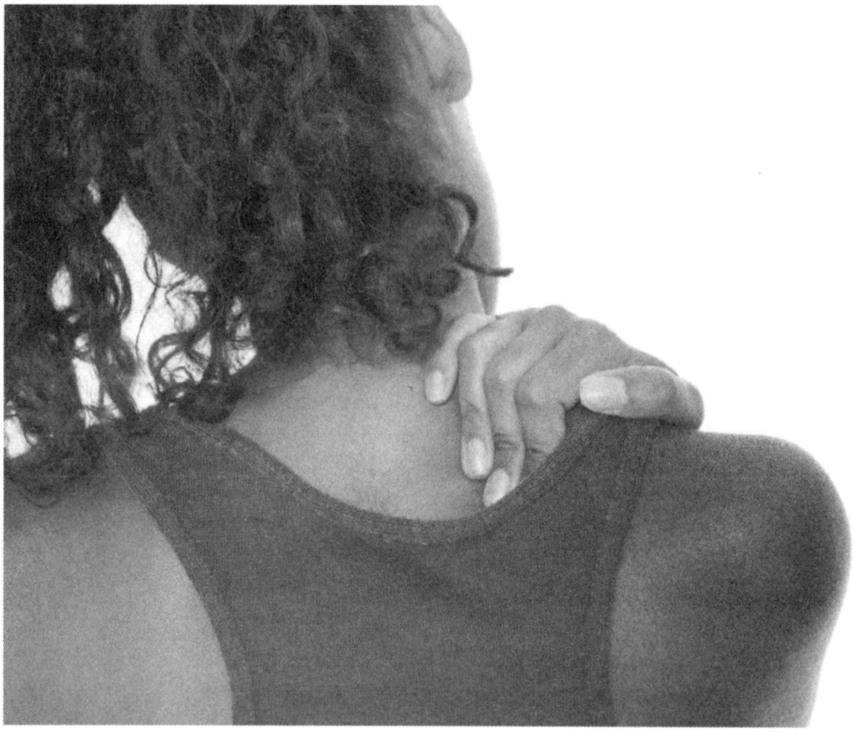

Fibromyalgia

Fibromyalgia (FM) affects an estimated 5 million Americans, 80%-90% of whom are women. The disorder is characterized by **widespread pain** and diffuse tenderness, but the disorder carries with it a number of other **life-disrupting symptoms** that vary from individual to individual. The exact causes of FM are not well understood, but hypothesized culprits include **traumatic** or **stressful life events** and **repetitive injuries.** Because there are no known biological markers, **diagnosing fibromyalgia** can be **problematic**.

Because medical treatment of fibromyalgia is not very effective, acupuncture is used by one in five fibromyalgia patients within two years of diagnosis.

Many clinical trials testing acupuncture for the treatment of FM were **inconclusive**, usually due to **small sample sizes** and **lack** of **sham** (placebo) control. These studies typically utilized a

standard protocol (as opposed to an **individualized protocol** which is how acupuncture is traditionally practiced) for each patient, which probably also contributed to the mixed results.

A recent study utilized **individualized acupuncture treatments** in patients with FM. Patients were diagnosed according to Traditional Chinese Medicine (TCM) theory and treated nine times. At the end of the study, the researchers concluded "Individualized acupuncture treatment in patients with fibromyalgia **proved efficacious** in terms of **pain relief** compared with placebo treatment. The effects persisted at **one year**, and its side effects were mild and infrequent" **("Acupuncture for Fibromyalgia in Primary Care: A Randomized Controlled Trial",** ***Acupunct Med*** **2016; 34: 257-266). http://aim.bmj.com/content/34/4/257**

Dive Deeper into Biomedicine- Potential Fibromyalgia Breakthrough

Research into acupuncture has often resulted in breakthroughs in other areas of medicine. Researchers studying the effects of acupuncture on FM patients found a **promising discovery**. They treated FM patients twice per week for one month (eight treatments), and found that acupuncture decreased FM pain, and it did it by increasing the activity of **pain-killing receptors** in the brain, while sham acupuncture did not.

They also noted that the reduction of pain was linked with reductions in **glutamate** (a neurotransmitter) levels in the brain. Patients with greater reductions in pain showed greater reductions in glutamate.

This suggests that glutamate may play a role in this disease and that it could potentially be used as a **biomarker** of disease severity **("Pain in Fibromyalgia is Linked to Changes in Brain Molecule",** ***University of Michigan Health System*****, March 13, 2008). https://www.sciencedaily.com/releases/2008/03/080310112658.htm**

Recommended Treatment Protocol: Physical exam and acupuncture twice per week for one month (eight treatments) is considered one course of treatment. Multiple courses may be necessary. **Each clinical scenario is different, and the acupuncture protocol will be individualized to the exact medical presentation.**

Treatment Goals: Reduce the intensity, frequency, and duration of fibromyalgia symptoms.

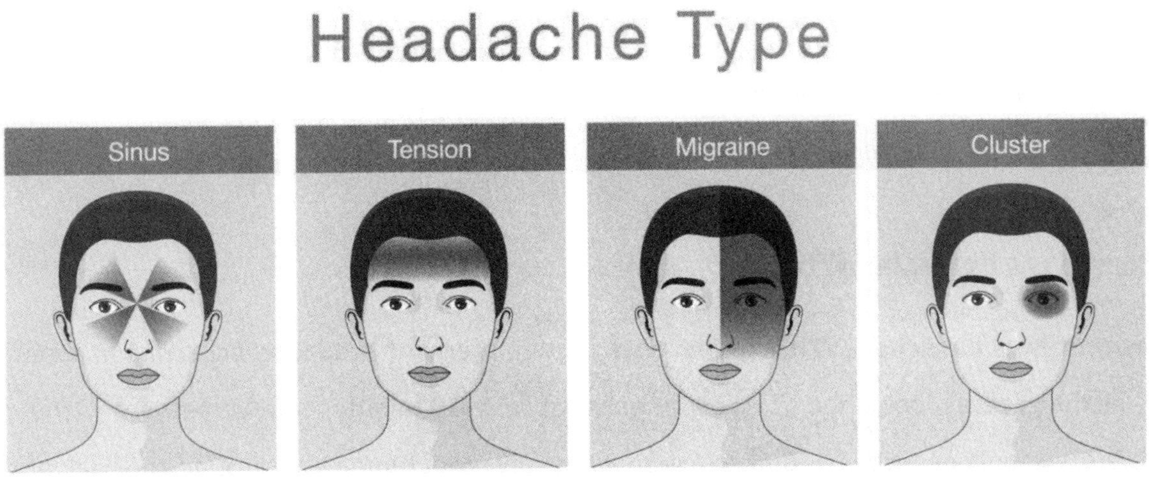

Headache

Headaches are among the most common medical complaints but the exact nature of headache pain remains unclear. Interestingly, the **brain** itself is not sensitive to pain because it lacks **pain receptors.** However, there are many pain-sensitive structures in the skull and neck, and these respond well to acupuncture treatment.

There are many **triggers** of headaches including: fatigue, sleep deprivation, side effects of medications or recreational drugs, dehydration, blood sugar disorders, viral infections, common cold, head injury, dental issues, sinus issues, stress, food allergies, hypertension, chemical exposure, and musculoskeletal disorders.

According to **The Acupuncture Evidence Project (www.acupuncture.org.au)**, there is strong evidence supporting the effectiveness of acupuncture for **headache** (chronic, tension-type, and migraine). Some headaches can be **completely eliminated** with acupuncture, while others can be **successfully managed** by reducing the frequency, intensity, and/or duration of headache pain. How well a patient responds to acupuncture depends on the clinical presentation. In the Traditional Chinese Medicine (TCM) model, all headaches are viewed as systemic problems and are treated with a **holistic** approach.

Tension Type Headache (TTH)

Tension-type headaches (TTH) are the most common form of headache, occurring in about 75% of the general population. TTH commonly last from 30 minutes to seven days, and the pain is commonly described as dull pain across the forehead, temples, or around the back of the head.

> **Cochrane Reviews** are systematic reviews of primary research in human health care and health policy, and are internationally recognized as the highest standard in evidence-based health care.

A **Cochrane Review** on acupuncture for tension type headaches was completed in 2016. After analyzing the data, the researchers concluded: "The available evidence suggests that a course of acupuncture consisting of **at least six treatment** sessions can be a **valuable option** for people with frequent tension type headaches". They also determined that how often patients got a TTH was **cut in half** and the effect of acupuncture was still present after **six months** **("Cochrane Review: Acupuncture for Tension Type Headaches, *Cochrane Database Syst Rev*, 2016 April 19). http://www.cochrane.org/CD007587/SYMPT_acupuncture-tension-type-headache**

Further, a study conducted in the United Kingdom concluded that "the **improvement in quality-adjusted-life-years** was achieved at a **very low cost** compared with routine medical treatment. Patients who received acupuncture had **22 fewer days** of headache, **15% lower** use of **medications**, and **25% fewer visits** to medical providers over one year compared to those who had usual medical care" **("Cost Effectiveness Analysis of a Randomized Trial of Acupuncture from Chronic Headache in Primary Care", *BMJ* 2004 Mar 27; 328(7442): 747). https://www.ncbi.nlm.nih.gov/pubmed/15023830**

Migraine

Migraine headache is a result of **specific changes** within the brain. It causes severe head pain that is often accompanied by sensitivity to light, sound, or smells. According to the **National Headache Foundation**, more than 37 million Americans suffer from migraine, and it affects three times as many women as men.

> **Cochrane Reviews** are systematic reviews of primary research in human health care and health policy, and are internationally recognized as the highest standard in evidence-based health care.

A **Cochrane Review** for the use of acupuncture for **treating** migraine was conducted in 2009. The researchers concluded "Available studies suggest that **acupuncture** is at least **as effective** as, or **possibly more effective** than, prophylactic drug treatment, and has **fewer adverse effects.** Acupuncture should be considered a **treatment option** for patients willing to undergo this treatment" **("Acupuncture for Migraine Prophylaxis",** ***Cochrane Database Syst Rev,*** **2009 Jan 21; (1):CD001218). https://www.ncbi.nlm.nih.gov/pubmed/19160193**

Another **Cochrane Review** on acupuncture for **preventing** migraine was conducted with similar results (acupuncture was **very effective** and **outperformed drugs**). Researchers concluded "The available evidence suggests that a course of acupuncture consisting of **at least six treatments** can be a **valuable option** for people with migraine". They also state the **frequency of migraine** for those receiving acupuncture was basically **cut in half** and people receiving acupuncture reported **less side effects** than people receiving drugs. **http://www.cochrane.org/CD001218/SYMPT_acupuncture-preventing-migraine-attacks**

Dive Deeper into Biomedicine- Acupuncture Regulates Nitric Oxide for Migraine Relief

One of the most amazing things about acupuncture is its ability to promote the **self-regulation** of the body. Sometimes there is too much of a good thing (in Traditional Chinese Medicine terms, this is referred to as an **"excess"** condition).

Nitric Oxide (NO) is a **signaling molecule** which regulates blood pressure, contributes to the immune response, controls neurotransmission and participates in cell differentiation and many more physiological functions.

In one study, nitric oxide (NO) levels were found to be **55% higher** in migraine patients compared to a control group. After **one** acupuncture treatment, migraine patients' NO levels **dropped 4.86%**, but after **five** acupuncture treatments, the NO levels of the migraine patients **dropped 30.63%**.

This not only shows that acupuncture promotes **self-regulation** in the body, but it also shows the **cumulative effect** of acupuncture treatments **("The Impact of Acupuncture Treatment on Nitric Oxide (NO) in Migraine Patients",** ***Acupunct Electrother Res,*** **2014; 39 (3-4):275-83). https://www.ncbi.nlm.nih.gov/pubmed/25693309**

Recommended Treatment Protocol: Physical Exam and eight treatments (2x/week for 4 weeks) is considered one course of treatment. Multiple courses of treatment may be necessary.

Treatment Goals: Determine causal factors of headache pain (if possible) and reduce the frequency, intensity, and duration of headache pain.

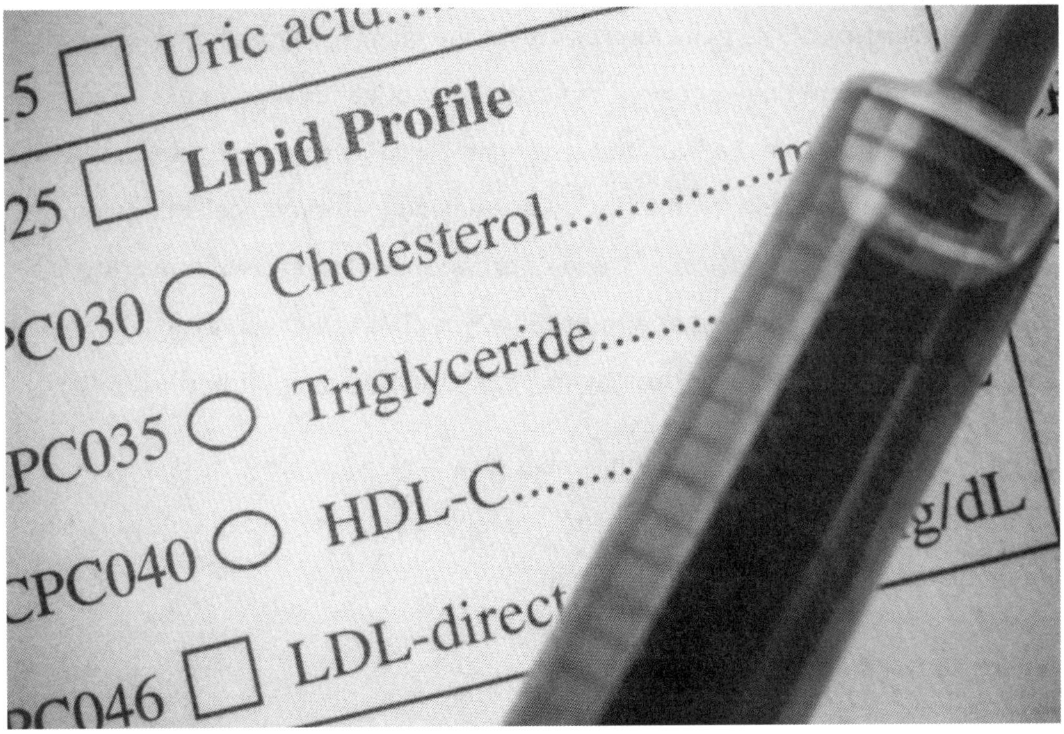

High Cholesterol

According to the **Mayo Clinic**, **cholesterol** is a waxy substance that's found in the **fats** (lipids) in your blood. While your body needs cholesterol to continue building healthy cells, having high cholesterol can increase your risk of heart disease. **(www.mayoclinic.org)**

It is important to note that **lifestyle factors** such as **exercise levels, nutritional status**, and **smoking** play significant roles in **heart disease.** While cholesterols role in heart disease is currently being debated, one thing is clear: altering your lifestyle is the single most important way of reducing the risk of heart disease.

For those who wish to lower their cholesterol levels, **electro-acupuncture** is a **safe** and **effective** drug-free option. Animal studies show electro-acupuncture (EA) at an acupoint traditionally used for fat loss (*Fenglong* ST40) **lowers lipid profiles** as well as the drug Simvastatin (without the dangerous side effects). It has been determined that the EA achieved this result by modulation of the **gene expression** in the rats. The global gene expression profile showed that EA not only regulated the expression of genes which were directly involved in **cholesterol metabolism** in the liver, but also significantly affected the **expression of genes** involved in **signal transduction**, **transcription regulation**, **cell cycle, cell adhesion, immunity**, and **stress ("Modulation of Gene Expression in Cholesterol Lowering Effect of Electro-Acupuncture at Fenglong Acupoint (ST40): a cDNA Microarray Study,** ***Int J Mol Med*** **2007 Apr; 19(4): 617-629). https://www.ncbi.nlm.nih.gov/pubmed/17334637**

Recommended Treatment Protocol: Physical exam and eight treatments (2x/week for four weeks) is considered one course of treatment. Multiple courses of treatment may be necessary. **Lifestyle modification is greatly encouraged.**

Treatment Goals: Lower risk of heart disease.

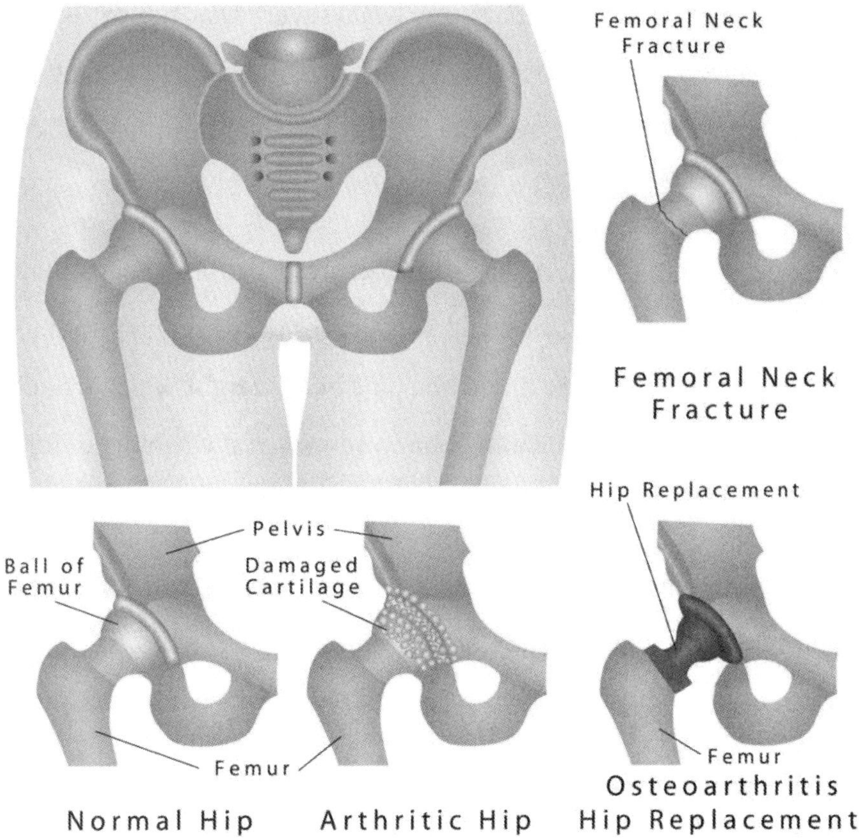

Hip: Hip Bursitis, Hip Degeneration, Hip Pain

Hip joints sustain **enormous stress** in daily activities such as walking. For example, during walking, when the left limb is lifted, the right hip joint is subjected to **compression forces several times greater** than the body weight. A person does not feel this huge force of compression because there are no nerves in the **articular cartilage.** When this cartilage is **eroded** by degenerative disease or aging, the bony head of the femur, which is richly supplied by sensory nerves, produces pain during every step because of this compressive force.

Hip bursitis (also called trochanteric bursitis) typically presents as pain over the affected bursa. The **bursa** is a small fluid filled sac that reduces friction between the moving parts of the hip.

When this **bursa** becomes **inflamed**, the pain may be so severe that the patient cannot lie on the affected side or even sit comfortably. Usually the patient feels pain during activity, but the pain can also vary. It can be local, right over the greater trochanter, in the iliac crest, or even in the knee region.

Hip bursitis can be treated very effectively by acupuncture because needling relaxes muscles, activates local anti-inflammatory reactions, and encourages tissue regeneration. However, it is important to note that unlike the upper limbs, the hips **bear weight** which makes them not only more susceptible to **degenerative change** but also makes the healing of injuries more difficult and **prolongs** the process of restoring normal physical function.

It should also be noted that underlying conditions causing **joint deformity** or **severe degeneration** will **reduce** the effectiveness of acupuncture.

Recommended Treatment Protocol: Physical Exam and eight treatments (2x/week for 4 weeks) is considered one course of treatment. Multiple courses of treatment may be necessary.

Treatment Goals: Reduce the frequency, intensity, and duration of hip pain, promote functional recovery of hip joint, and to eliminate, reduce or delay the need for hip replacement surgery.

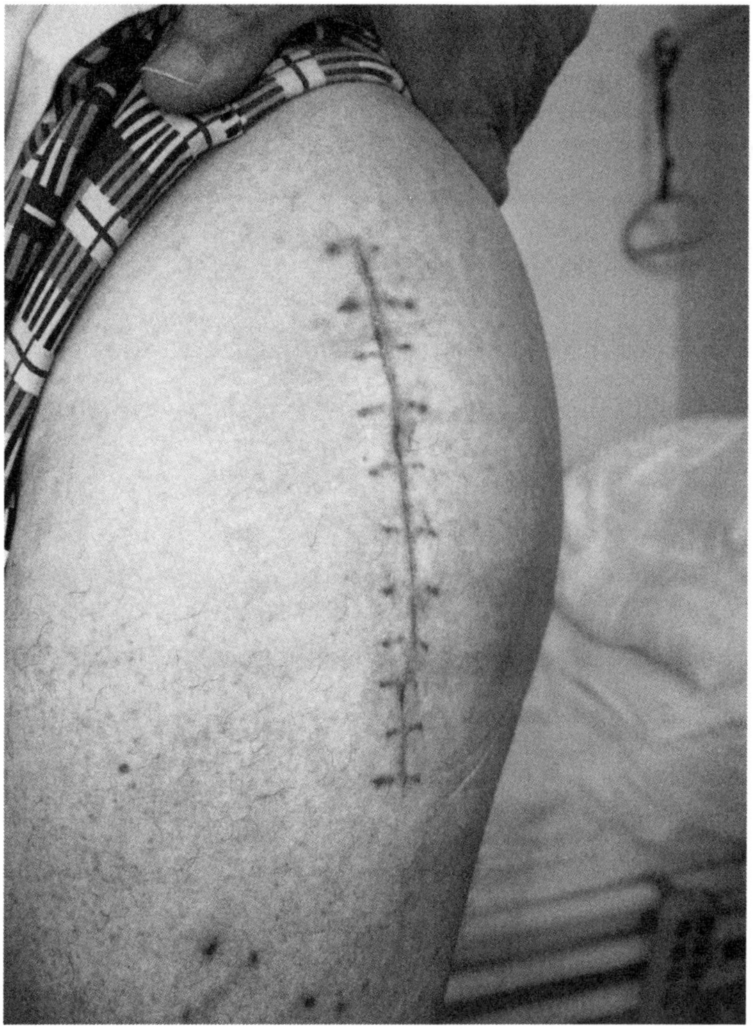

Hip: Post Replacement Surgery Recovery

When all other therapies have failed surgery may be necessary to relieve pain and restore function to the hip. The number of total hip replacement surgeries performed in the U.S. has increased substantially over the last 10 years, and has become much more common in younger people.

However, it may be **months** following surgery before the patient is fully healed, and the patient may suffer significantly throughout the recovery period.

Nerves heal at a slow rate, approximately one millimeter per day (about one inch per month). Recent studies demonstrate that "**acupuncture** significantly improves **motor nerve conduction velocity** and **amplitude** and also promotes **functional nerve repair**" **(*Neural Regeneration Research* V10, no. 1 (2015): 128).**
https://www.ncbi.nlm.nih.gov/pmc/articles/PMC4357096/

Further, acupuncture accelerates **recovery** after **general anesthesia ("Acupuncture Accelerates Recovery after General Anesthesia: A Prospective Randomized Controlled Trial", *J Integr Med.* 2015 Mar; 13(2): 99-104).**
https://www.ncbi.nlm.nih.gov/pubmed/25797640

And finally, according to the **Center for Disease Control (CDC)**, smokers have lower survival rates after surgery and greater risk for complications. If a smoker is considering a surgery, it is imperative that they **quit smoking**.
https://www.cdc.gov/tobacco/data_statistics/sgr/2004/highlights/other_effects/index.htm

For more information on the importance of quitting smoking and how acupuncture can assist in this process, see **"Stop Smoking"**.

Follow all instructions and restrictions provided by your surgeon. The length of time your restrictions are in place is determined by your surgeon and how quickly you heal. Clinically, acupuncture and electro-acupuncture can significantly shorten the recovery process and result in improved outcomes including the reduction of possible complications.

For best results, it is best to start acupuncture as soon after the surgical procedure as realistically possible.

Recommended Treatment Protocol: Physical Exam and twelve treatments (2x/week for 6 weeks) is considered one course of treatment. Multiple courses of treatment may be necessary.

Treatment Goals: Reduce pain and recovery time, and increase functional recovery of the hip.

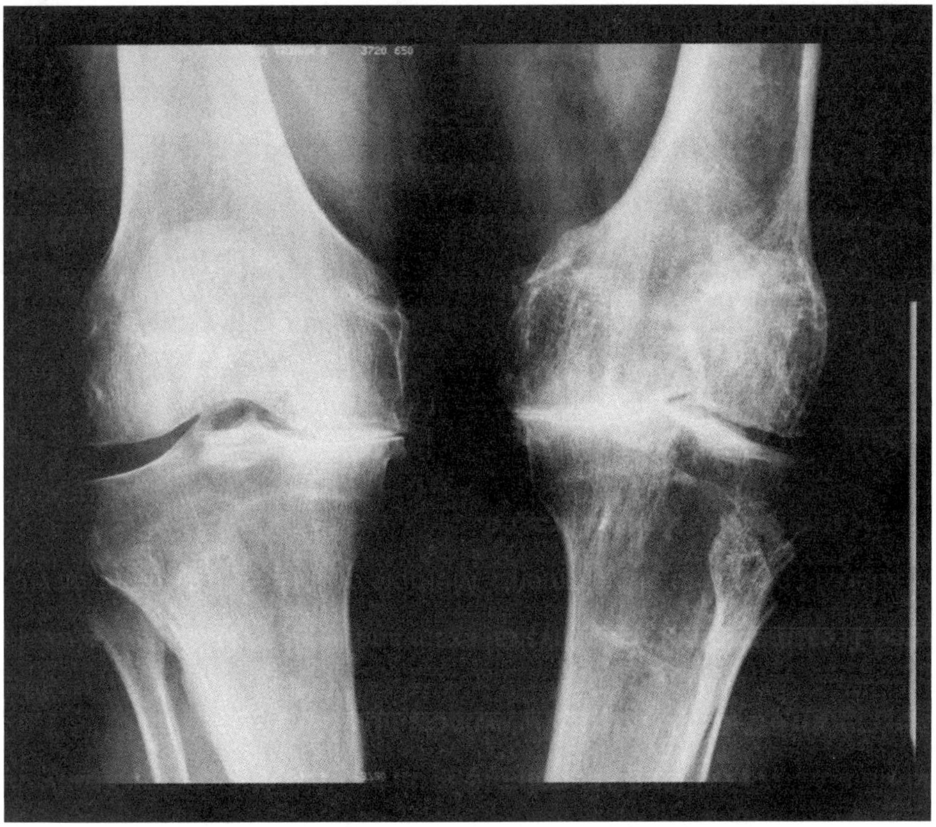

Knee: Knee Pain/Osteoarthritis/Knee Strain

Everyday activities such as walking, climbing stairs, or rising from a chair, as well as athletic activities such as running and jumping, depend on the **functional integrity** of the knee. Any diseases or trauma to the bone or soft tissues can significantly impair the knee's ability to perform basic functions.

Knee pain is usually caused by **degenerative changes**, **inflammation, traumatic injury**, **infections,** or **referred pain** from **hip** or **spine disorders**. Knee pain is commonly seen clinically, and acupuncture is very effective in restoring functional integrity of the knee.

In multiple studies, acupuncture has also been found to be an effective treatment for pain and physical dysfunction associated with **osteoarthritis** of the knee **("Acupuncture and Osteoarthritis of the Knee: A Review of Randomized, Controlled Trials", *Fam Community Health,* 2008Jul-Sept;31(3):247-254) https://www.ncbi.nlm.nih.gov/pmc/articles/PMC2810544/ , ("The Effect of Acupuncture on the Symptoms of Knee Osteoarthritis- An Open Randomized Controlled Study", *Acupunct Med* 2004, Mar; 22(1):14-22). https://www.ncbi.nlm.nih.gov/pubmed/15077933**

Dive Deeper into Biomedicine- Cortisone Injections Damage Cartilage

Cortisone Injections are commonly given for knee pain. They reduce inflammation and reduce pain in some cases. However, a 2017 **JAMA** study shows that outcomes for cortisone injections are **no better than placebo** (saline) injections for pain, and the cortisone injections had **worse** long term outcomes: at **two years** the cortisone group had **twice** as much **cartilage loss** vs the saline injection group, and the cortisone group had a higher **arthritis index score** as well **("Effect of Intra-Articular Triamcinolone vs Saline on Knee Cartilage Volume and Pain in Patients with Knee Osteoarthritis", *JAMA* 2017;317(19):1967-1975). https://jamanetwork.com/journals/jama/article-abstract/2626573**

A **PDF** of the full study can be found here: **http://preview.thenewsmarket.com/Previews/JOUR/DocumentAssets/472612.pdf**

Recommended Treatment Protocol: Physical Exam and eight treatments (2x/week for 4 weeks) is considered one course of treatment. Multiple courses of treatment may be necessary.

Treatment Goals: Reduce the frequency, intensity, and duration of knee pain, and promote functional recovery of the knee.

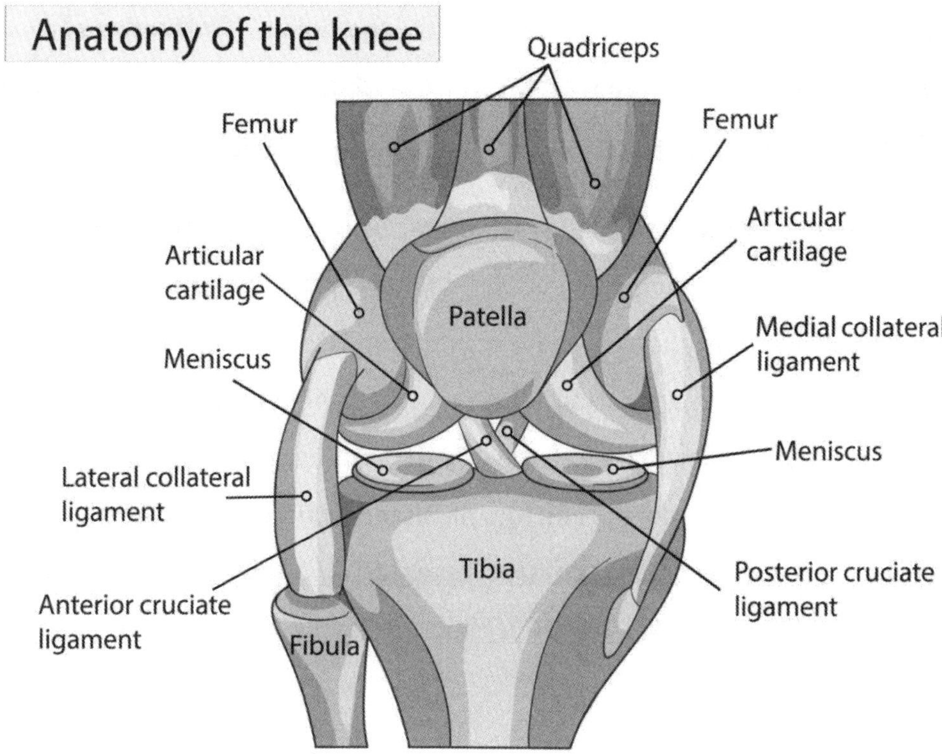

Knee: Medial or Lateral Meniscus Injury/ ACL/PCL Injury/Patellar Bursitis

Everyday activities such as walking, climbing stairs, or rising from a chair, as well as athletic activities such as running and jumping, depend on the **functional integrity** of the knee. **Trauma** to the bone or soft tissues can significantly impair the knee's ability to perform basic functions. In the early phases, a patient may feel knee **weakness** rather than pain.

Acupuncture is commonly used to reduce pain and promote healing. Researchers compared the effectiveness of acupuncture to physical therapy in a 2016 study. After analyzing their results, they concluded "These results indicate that acupuncture represents a certain clinical effect on knee **osteoarthritis** which is superior compared to **physiotherapy** (physical therapy), and hint at the possible roles of acupuncture in promoting **cartilage** repair" **("Influence of Acupuncture in Treating Knee Osteoarthritis and Cartilage Repairing",** ***Am J Transl Res,*** **2016; 8(9): 3995-4002). https://www.ncbi.nlm.nih.gov/pmc/articles/PMC5040698/**

Electro-Acupuncture can **reduce pain** and **inflammation**, and significantly improve the **healing** of **soft tissues**. An amazing study published in the journal ***Stem Cells*** in 2017 showed that electro-acupuncture in rats, horses, and humans stimulated and mobilized **mesenchymal stem cells (MSC)** into systemic circulation. This resulted in **higher thresholds** for injury-induced **pain** and considerably increased a type of **collagen** that promotes tendon **repair** and **anti-inflammatory** cells known to be predictors of **faster healing time (*Stem Cell* 2017; 35; 1303-1315). https://www.sciencedaily.com/releases/2017/03/170316174225.htm http://onlinelibrary.wiley.com/doi/10.1002/stem.2613/full**

Dive Deeper into Biomedicine- Common Medical Procedures for Knee Conditions

<u>**Cortisone Injections-**</u> **Cortisone Injections** are commonly given for knee pain. They reduce inflammation and reduce pain in some cases. However, a 2017 **JAMA** study shows outcomes for cortisone injections are **no better than placebo** (saline) for pain, and cortisone injections had **worse** long term outcomes: after **two years** the cortisone group had <u>**twice**</u> as much **cartilage loss** compared to the saline injection group, and the cortisone group had a higher **arthritis index** score as well **("Effect of Intra-Articular Triamcinolone vs Saline on Knee Cartilage Volume and Pain in Patients with Knee Osteoarthritis", *JAMA* 2017; 317(19): 1967-1975).** <u>**https://jamanetwork.com/journals/jama/article-abstract/2626573**</u>

A **PDF** of the full study can be found here: <u>**http://preview.thenewsmarket.com/Previews/JOUR/DocumentAssets/472612.pdf**</u>

<u>**Arthroscopic Knee Surgery-**</u> **Arthroscopic knee surgery (meniscestomy)** is the **most common procedure** done in the **world,** and 700,000 are performed in the U.S. every year. However, several studies have shown that they are <u>**no better than placebo**</u> surgeries:

"Why Do Surgeons Continue to Perform Unnecessary Surgery?", *Patient Safety in Surgery*, 2017, 11:1 <u>**https://pssjournal.biomedcentral.com/articles/10.1186/s13037-016-0117-6,**</u>

"Four Orthopedic Surgeries No Better than Placebo", *Pain Science*, March 3, 2017 <u>**https://www.painscience.com/biblio/four-orthopedic-surgeries-no-better-than-placebo.html**</u>

<u>**Recommended Treatment Protocol:**</u> Physical Exam and twelve treatments (2x/week for 6 weeks) is considered one course of treatment. Multiple courses may be necessary.

<u>**Treatment Goals**</u>**:** Reduce the frequency, intensity, and duration of knee pain, and to promote functional recovery of the knee.

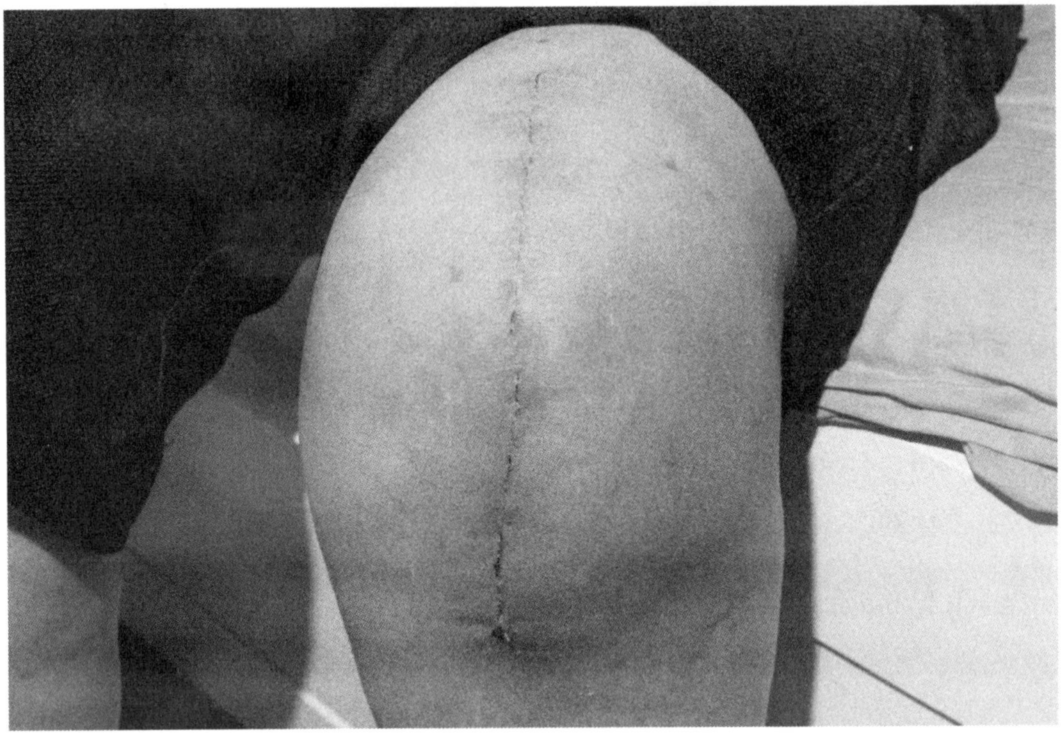

Knee: Post Knee Replacement Surgery Recovery

When all other therapies have failed **surgery** may be necessary to relieve pain and restore function to the knee. The number of total **knee replacement surgeries** performed in the U.S. **increased 93%** between 2001 and 2011, and it is expected to increase to 3.48 million surgeries annually by 2030.

However, it may be **months** following surgery before the patient is fully healed, and the patient may suffer significantly throughout the recovery period.

Nerves heal at a slow rate, approximately one millimeter per day (about one inch per month). Recent studies demonstrate that "**acupuncture** significantly **improves motor nerve conduction velocit**y and **amplitude** and also promotes **functional nerve repair**" (***Neural***

***Regeneration Research* V10, no. 1 (2015): 128).**
https://www.ncbi.nlm.nih.gov/pmc/articles/PMC4357096/

Further, **acupuncture** accelerates **recovery** after **general anesthesia ("Acupuncture Accelerates Recovery after General Anesthesia: A Prospective Randomized Controlled Trial", *J Integr Med.* 2015 Mar; 13(2): 99-104).**
https://www.ncbi.nlm.nih.gov/pubmed/25797640

And finally, according to the **Centers for Disease Control (CDC)**, smokers have **lower survival rates** after surgery and **greater risk** for **complications**. If a smoker is considering any surgery, it is imperative that they **quit smoking**.
https://www.cdc.gov/tobacco/data_statistics/sgr/2004/highlights/other_effects/index.htm

For more information on the importance of quitting smoking and how acupuncture can assist in this process, see **"Stop Smoking"**.

After a knee replacement surgery, follow all instructions and restrictions provided by your surgeon. The length of time your restrictions are in place is determined by your surgeon and how quickly you heal. Acupuncture and electro-acupuncture can significantly shorten the recovery process and result in improved outcomes including the reduction of possible complications. For best results, it is best to start acupuncture as soon after the surgical procedure as realistically possible.

Recommended Treatment Protocol: Physical Exam and twelve treatments (2x/week for 6 weeks) is considered one course of treatment. Multiple courses may be necessary.

Treatment Goals: Reduce pain and recovery time, and increase functional recovery of the knee.

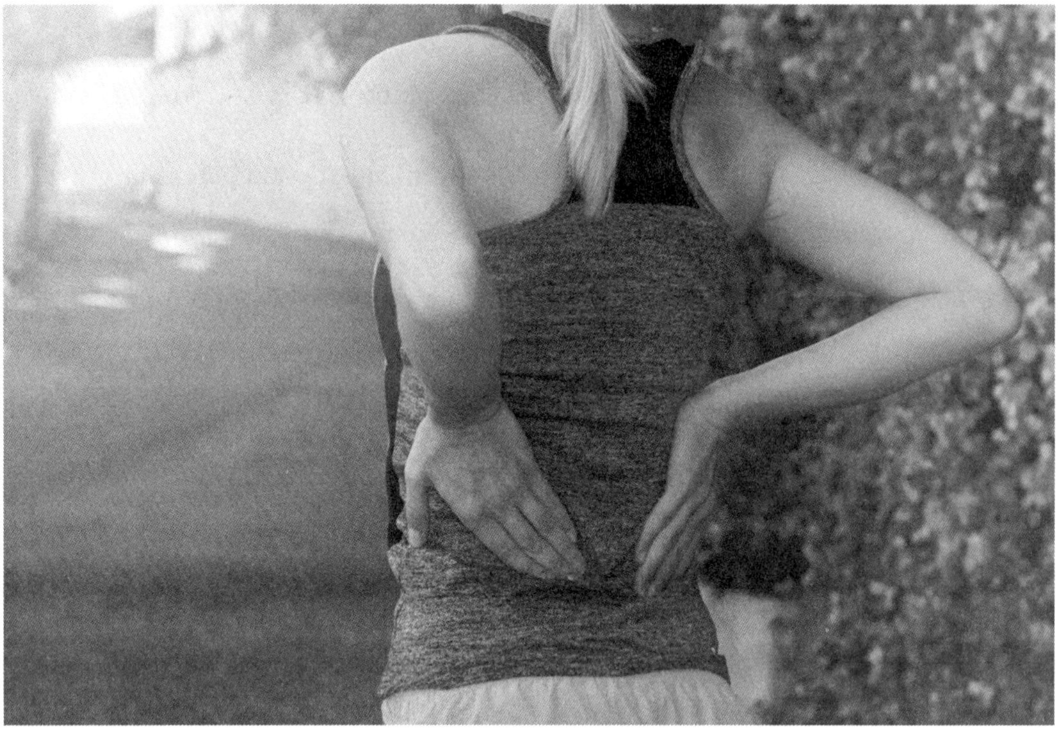

Low Back: General Pain/Sprain

Low back pain is one of the **most common** problems seen in the United States. Statistics show that about 150 million Americans suffer from **acute** or **chronic** low back pain. **Common causes** of low back pain include improper lifting, poor posture, lack of regular exercise, overuse, and being overweight. Other causes include arthritis, fracture, degeneration, and herniated intervertebral discs.

Medications are commonly used to **manage** low back pain, but both over the counter and prescription medications have been shown to only provide **limited relief** and also have **unwanted side effects,** some of them severe. **Luckily, most musculoskeletal disorders respond very well to acupuncture therapy.**

Research has confirmed what the Chinese knew 2,000 years ago- acupuncture is very useful for conditions like chronic low back pain **("Acupuncture for Low Back Pain: An Overview of Systematic Reviews",** ***Evid Based Alternat Med*** **2015;2015:328196).**
https://www.ncbi.nlm.nih.gov/pmc/articles/PMC4364128/

In 2017 the **American College of Physicians (ACP)** issued a "**strong recommendation**" of using acupuncture as a **first line therapy** for the treatment of low back pain that does not radiate down the leg **("Noninvasive Treatments for Acute, Subacute, and Chronic Low Back Pain: A Clinical Practice Guideline from the American College of Physicians",** ***Annals of Internal Medicine*****, Clinical Guidelines, 4 April 2017).**
http://annals.org/aim/article/2603228/noninvasive-treatments-acute-subacute-chronic-low-back-pain-clinical-practice

For chronic low back pain, bed rest should be avoided. For chronic low back pain, or any chronic pain for that matter, it is important to get moving as much as possible as soon as possible.

Recommended Treatment Protocol: Physical Exam and eight treatments (2x/week for 4 weeks) is considered one course of treatment. Multiple courses may be necessary.

Treatment Goals: Reduce the frequency, intensity, and duration of low back pain.

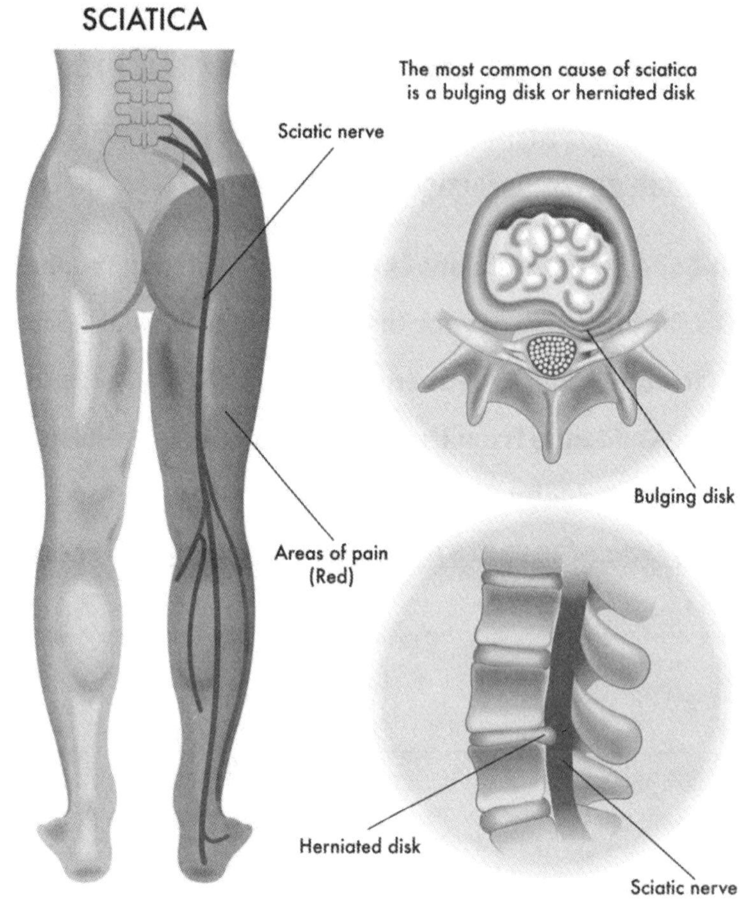

Low Back: Lumbar Herniated Nucleus Prolapse (HNP) Pain/Herniated Disc/Bulging Disc/Sciatica/Degenerative Disc Disease/Degenerative Joint Disease/Stenosis Pain

Herniated discs, bulging disc, slipped disc, herniated nucleus pulposus (HNP)- Spinal discs are soft, compressible discs that **separate interlocking bones** (vertebrae) that make up the spine. These discs act as **shock absorbers** for the spine, allowing it to flex, bend, and twist. Bulging, herniated or ruptured discs can occur when the intervertebral discs become compressed and **bulge outward** (herniate) or **rupture**, causing **nerve irritation**.

Sciatica – **Sciatica** is caused by **compression** of the **sciatic nerve**, the large nerve that travels through the buttocks and extends down the back of the leg. This compression causes shock-like or burning low back pain combined with pain through the buttocks and down one leg, occasionally reaching the foot. In extreme cases, the symptoms may involve not only **pain** but **numbness** and **muscle weakness** in the leg because of **interrupted nerve signaling**.

Degenerative Disc Disease (DDD)- **Degenerative disc disease** is a term used to describe the age-related changes in the discs.

Degenerative Joint Disease (DJD)- **Degenerative joint disease** is also known as **osteoarthritis** and is caused by the inflammation, breakdown, and eventual loss of **cartilage** of the joints.

Stenosis- **Stenosis** is a narrowing of the **spinal column** that puts **pressure** on the **spinal cord** and **nerves** that can cause pain or numbness with walking and over time leads to leg weakness and sensory loss.

A wide range of medications are used to treat low back pain, both **over the counter (OTC)** and **prescription**. The **risks** of these drugs include **interactions** with other medications and the possibility of **side effects,** including liver damage, gastrointestinal bleeding, heart damage, kidney damage, and addiction. In fact, because of the **misuse** of powerful pain medications, the U.S. is currently experiencing a public health crisis known as the **"opioid epidemic"**.

According to the **National Institute of Health's National Institute of Drug Abuse**, in the late 1990's **pharmaceutical companies** reassured the medical community that patients would not become addicted to prescription opioid pain relievers, and healthcare providers began to prescribe them at greater rates. This subsequently led to widespread misuse of these medications before it became clear that these medications could indeed be **highly addictive**. Now, **every day**, more than **90 Americans die** after overdosing on opioids and the economic burden of prescription opioid misuse in the U.S. is $78.5 billion a year **(www.drugabuse.gov)**.

Acupuncture can play a large role in helping to address this crisis, and several large acupuncture organizations have written white papers on the **evidence**, **cost-effectiveness,** and **care availability** for acupuncture as a primary, non-pharmacologic method for **pain management**. **http://www.nccaom.org/wp-content/uploads/pdf/Acupunctures%20Role%20in%20Solving%20the%20Opioid%20Epidemic2017.pdf**

Acupuncture has even been shown to be **more effective** than opioids for sciatica **("Comparative Clinical Effectiveness of Management Strategies for Sciatica: Systematic Review and Network Meta-Analysis",** ***Spine J.*** **2015 Jun 1; 15(6):1461-77). https://www.ncbi.nlm.nih.gov/pubmed/24412033**

When drug options fail, many people turn to surgery but these procedures are not always successful, have potential **complication**s, and can cause other problems such as **permanent** lack of flexibility and more pain, and there is **little evidence** to show what procedures work best for each patient's medical scenario.

In fact, data from clinical trials suggest that patients who have herniated lumbar discs have **similar long-term outcomes** whether they undergo **surgery** or elect **conservative management**. In addition, **contrary to what surgeons will tell you**, the **risk** of subsequent catastrophic worsening without surgery is **minimal** **(Resolution of Lumbar Disc Herniation without Surgery,** ***New England Journal of Medicine,*** **April 2016). http://www.nejm.org/doi/full/10.1056/NEJMicm1511194#t=article**

Lumbar disc herniation, like all spinal herniation, can fully heal and resolve. In fact, there are many **published case reports** of this occurring:

"Spontaneous Regression of Lumbar Herniated Discs: Report of One Illustrative Case and Review of the Literature" ***Clin Neurol Neurosurg*** **2016 Apr. 143: 86-89.** **https://www.ncbi.nlm.nih.gov/pubmed/26907997**

"Spontaneous Remission of a Big Subligamentous Extruded Disc Herniation: Case Report and Review of the Literature" ***Korean J Spine*** **2015 Mar; 12(1): 19-21).** **https://www.ncbi.nlm.nih.gov/pubmed/25883664**

Acupuncture can **promote** the **healing** of a **herniated disc**. In one published case report, a patient had a large lumbar disc herniation (confirmed by MRI) with radiating pain for two years. Two courses of physical therapy provided no relief and she could not take NSAIDS due to drug-induced gastric bleeding. She was referred to a surgeon, but did not want lumbar surgery. Instead she chose to try acupuncture.

Acupuncture was given twice per week for seven weeks, and the results were excellent. The patient was **pain free** and **continued** to be pain free at a **three month** follow up. Further, a follow up MRI showed considerable improvement **("Lumbar Disc Herniation Treated with Auricular Acupuncture: Why the(y) Wait?"** ***BMJ Acupuncture in Medicine,*** **V32, Issue 5).** **http://aim.bmj.com/content/32/5/430**

Smoking has been shown to **promote** the development of **lumbar herniation ("Is Smoking a Risk Factor for Lumbar Disc Herniation"?,** ***Eur Spine J*** **2016 Jan; 25(1): 168-76).** **https://www.ncbi.nlm.nih.gov/pubmed/26160690**

See **"Stop Smoking"** for more information on the importance of **quitting smoking** and how acupuncture can assist in this process.

> Acupuncture can help many patients with herniated discs and/or sciatica to experience a reduction of their pain and muscle spasms and resume normal work and lifestyle for years.

Recommended Treatment Protocol: Physical Exam and twelve treatments (2x/week for 6 weeks) is considered one course of treatment. Multiple courses of treatment may be necessary.

Treatment Goals: Reduce the frequency, intensity, and duration of low back pain, promote functional improvement and quality of life.

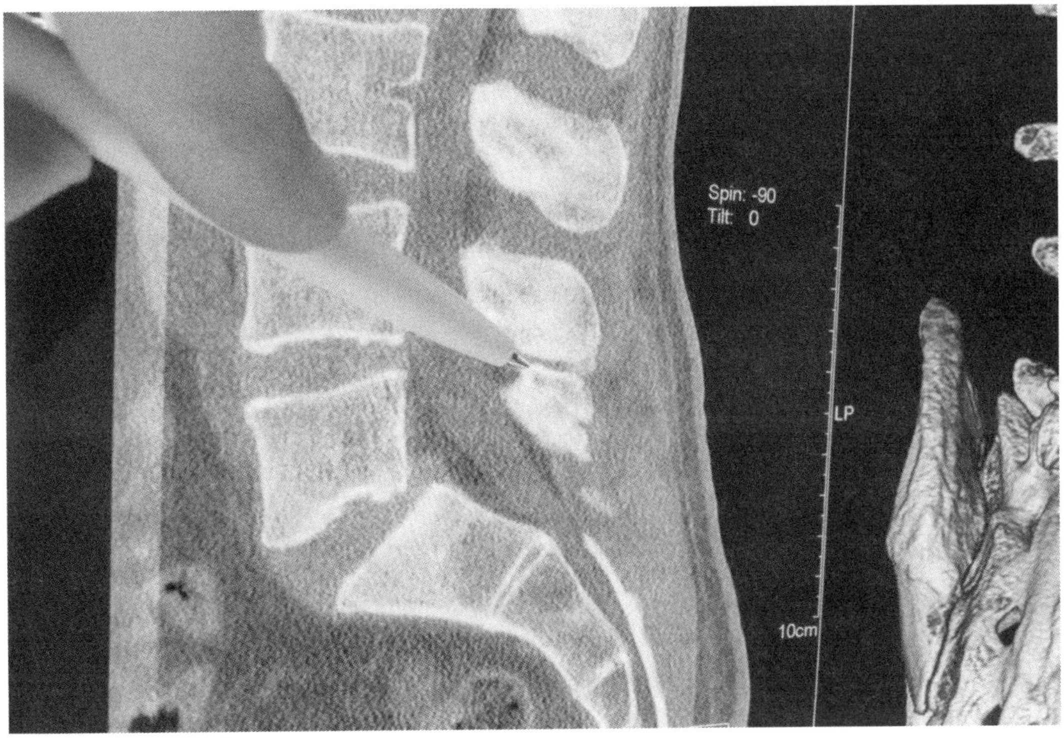

Lumbar MRI Guidelines

Although they are **commonly done**, medical guidelines actually **strongly discourage** the use of MRI and x-ray for **diagnosing low back pain** because they produce so many false alarms **("MRI and X-Ray Often Worse than Useless for Back pain", *Pain Science,* June 2, 2017).** **https://www.painscience.com/articles/mri-and-x-ray-almost-useless-for-back-pain.php**

Further, the **American College of Physicians (ACP)** has recommended **against** MRI and x-ray for the **diagnosis** of **low back pain** since **2007** **http://annals.org/aim/article/736814/diagnosis-treatment-low-back-pain-joint-clinical-practice-guideline-from** and **reinforced** their position in a **2011** review. **http://annals.org/aim/article/746774/diagnostic-imaging-low-back-pain-advice-high-value-health-care**

The reason that MRI and x-ray are **not recommended** for diagnosis of back pain is because **many people with no symptoms** **of back pain have disc degeneration, bulges, and other**

abnormalities on MRI. This calls into **question** the **relationship** between abnormalities seen on MRI and back pain in general.

Researchers conducting a review of studies on MRI finding of **asymptomatic people** (people with no symptoms of back pain) have questioned the value of MRI for diagnosing back pain, stating "Imaging findings of spine degeneration are present in high proportions of asymptomatic individuals, increasing with age." **("Systematic Literature Review of Imaging Features of Spinal Degeneration in Asymptomatic Populations",** ***Spine*****, Nov 27, 2014). https://www.ncbi.nlm.nih.gov/pubmed/25430861**

As the following table shows, 50% of all year 40 year-old people with no back pain have bulging disc(s) on MRI:

Table 2: Age Specific Prevalence Estimates of Degenerative Spine Imaging Findings in Asymptomatic (Pain Free) Patients **("Systematic Literature Review of Imaging Features of Spinal Degeneration in Asymptomatic Populations",** ***Spine*****, Nov 27, 2014). https://www.ncbi.nlm.nih.gov/pubmed/25430861**

			Age				
Finding	20	30	40	50	60	70	80
Disc degeneration	37%	52%	68%	80%	88%	93%	96%
Disc signal loss	17%	33%	54%	73%	86%	94%	97%
Disc height loss	24%	34%	45%	56%	67%	76%	84%
Disc bulge	30%	40%	50%	60%	69%	77%	84%
Disc protrusion	29%	31%	33%	36%	38%	40%	43%
Annular fissure	19%	20%	22%	23%	25%	27%	29%
Facet degeneration	4%	9%	18%	32%	50%	69%	83%
Spondylolisthesis	3%	5%	8%	14%	23%	35%	50%

The problem of connecting MRI findings to low back pain is compounded by the fact that MRI's are used in **clinical decision making** regarding **surgical procedures**. Patients may possibly be receiving surgeries that are **not necessary**.

In addition, **one should <u>always</u> get a second opinion regarding any surgery**, especially a **<u>spinal surgery</u>**. A 2013 study of spine surgery second opinions showed that of 183 second opinions seen over 20 months, the second opinion surgeon documented that the previous spine surgeon recommended an **"unnecessary"** surgery **60.7%** of the time, the **"wrong"** surgery **33.3%** of the time, and the **"right"** surgery **6%** of the time **("Are Recommended Spine Operations Either Unnecessary or Too Complex? Evidence from Second Opinions",** ***Surg Neurol Int.,*** **2013; 4 (Suppl 5); S353-S358).**
<u>https://www.ncbi.nlm.nih.gov/pmc/articles/PMC3841934/</u>

Dive Deeper into Biomedicine- Lumbar Surgeries to Avoid

All surgeries involve **risk**, and **several** surgical procedures that are promoted to reduce low back pain have been shown to be **ineffective**. These include:

Vertebroplasty for osteoporic compression fractures (stabilizing crushed vertebra) **("Four Orthopedic Surgeries No Better than Placebo",** ***Pain Science,*** **March 3, 2017).** **https://www.painscience.com/biblio/four-orthopedic-surgeries-no-better-than-placebo.html**

Spinal fusion **("Why Do Surgeons Continue to Perform Unnecessary surgery?",** ***Patient Safety in Surgery,*** **2017, 11:1).** **https://pssjournal.biomedcentral.com/articles/10.1186/s13037-016-0117-6**

Intradiscal electrothermal therapy (burning nerve fibers) **("Four Orthopedic Surgeries No Better than Placebo",** ***Pain Science,*** **March 3, 2017).** **https://www.painscience.com/biblio/four-orthopedic-surgeries-no-better-than-placebo.html**

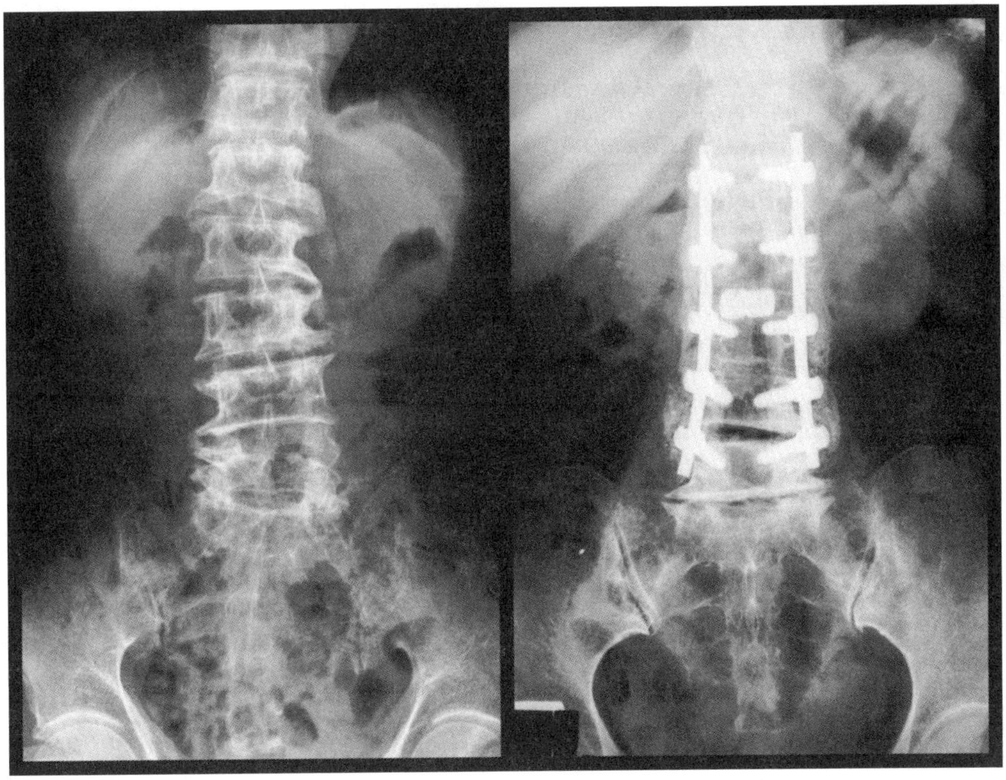

Low Back: Post Low Back Surgery Recovery

When all other therapies have failed surgery may be necessary to relieve pain caused by serious musculoskeletal injuries or nerve compression. However, it may be **months** following surgery before the patient is fully healed, and the patient may suffer significantly throughout the recovery period. Nerves heal at a slow rate, approximately one millimeter per day (about one inch per month). Recent studies demonstrate that "**acupuncture** significantly improves **motor nerve conduction velocity** and **amplitude** and also promotes **functional nerve repair**" **(*Neural Regeneration Research* V10, no. 1 (2015): 128).** **https://www.ncbi.nlm.nih.gov/pmc/articles/PMC4357096/**

Further, **acupunctur**e accelerates **recovery** after **general anesthesia ("Acupuncture Accelerates Recovery after General Anesthesia: A Prospective Randomized Controlled Trial",** ***J Integr Med.*** **2015 Mar; 13(2): 99-104).**
https://www.ncbi.nlm.nih.gov/pubmed/25797640

Follow all instructions and restrictions provided by your surgeon. The length of time your restrictions are in place is determined on your type of surgery. Generally speaking, it is best to start acupuncture as soon after the surgical procedure as realistically possible.

Acupuncture assists many patients with lumbar surgery to recover and to experience a reduction of their pain and muscle spasms and resume normal work and lifestyle for years.

And finally, according to the **Centers for Disease Control (CDC)**, smokers have **lower survival rates** after surgery and **greater risk** for complications. If a smoker is considering any surgery, it is imperative that they **quit smoking**.
https://www.cdc.gov/tobacco/data_statistics/sgr/2004/highlights/other_effects/index.htm

For more information on the importance of quitting smoking and how acupuncture can assist in this process, see **"Stop Smoking"**.

Recommended Treatment Protocol: Physical Exam and twelve treatments (2x/week for 6 weeks) consists of one course of treatment. Multiple courses of treatment may be necessary.

Treatment Goals: Reduce pain and increase functional recovery following lumbar surgery.

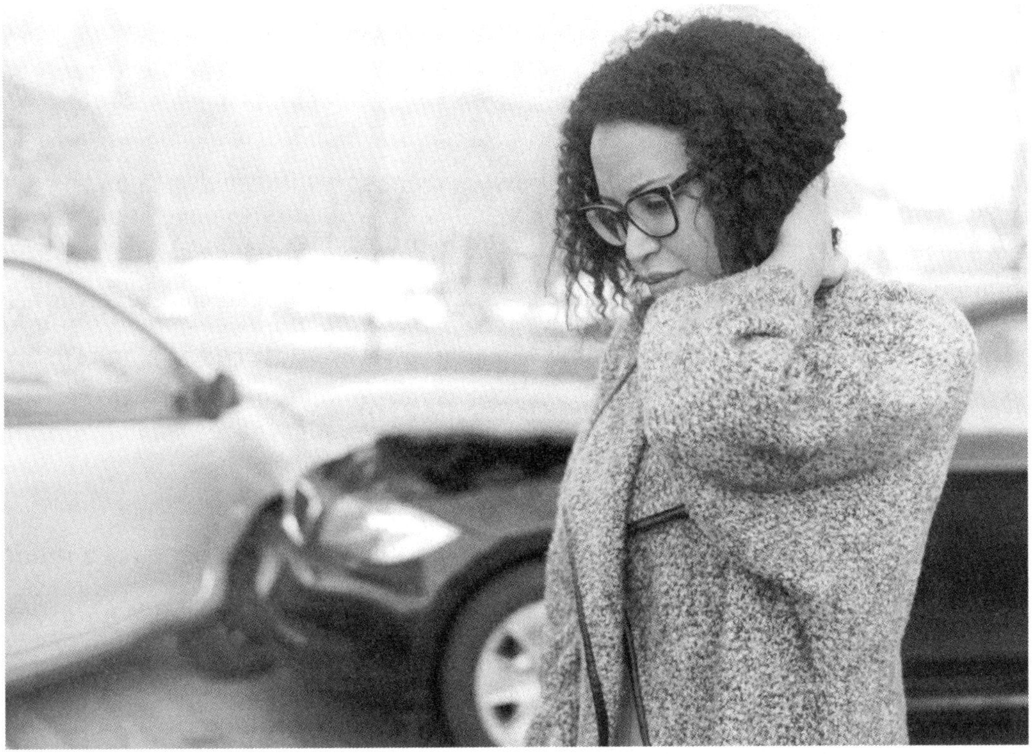

Neck: Cervical Sprain/Strain/Whiplash

The **neck** serves two basic functions: 1) as a passageway for blood, nerves, food, and air, and 2) as a pedestal to support the head. About two dozen muscles in the neck and upper back support and move the head and neck, and many important structures are crowded into this area as well. **Neck pain** can come from **bad posture** during work-related activities, improper **sleeping** position, or it can be caused by **cumulative trauma** from **frequent repetitions** of the same activity, **sports injuries**, or **car accidents**.

Sprain, strain, fatigue, inflammation, low circulation, or other injuries can cause weakness and tightness in one or more major muscle groups, causing the discs and joints to support more weight than they should, which in turn leads to chronic pain and premature degeneration.

Cochrane Reviews are systematic reviews of primary research in human health care and health policy, and are internationally recognized as the gold standard in evidence-based health care.

A **Cochrane Review** in 2006 summarized the most current scientific evidence on the effectiveness of acupuncture for acute, subacute, and chronic neck pain. After analyzing the data, the researchers concluded "There is moderate evidence that those that received acupuncture reported less pain at short term follow up" **("Acupuncture for Neck Disorders", *Cochrane Database Syst Rev*, 2006 Jul 19; (3): CD004870). https://www.ncbi.nlm.nih.gov/pubmed/16856065**

Acupuncture has been shown to help many patients with neck pain to experience a reduction of pain (frequency, duration, and intensity), reduce flare ups, slow degeneration, and resume normal work and lifestyle for years.

Recommended Treatment Protocol: Physical Exam and eight treatments (2x/week for 4 weeks) is considered one course of treatment. Multiple courses of treatment may be necessary.

Treatment Goals: Reduce the frequency, intensity, and duration of neck pain, promote functional improvement and quality of life.

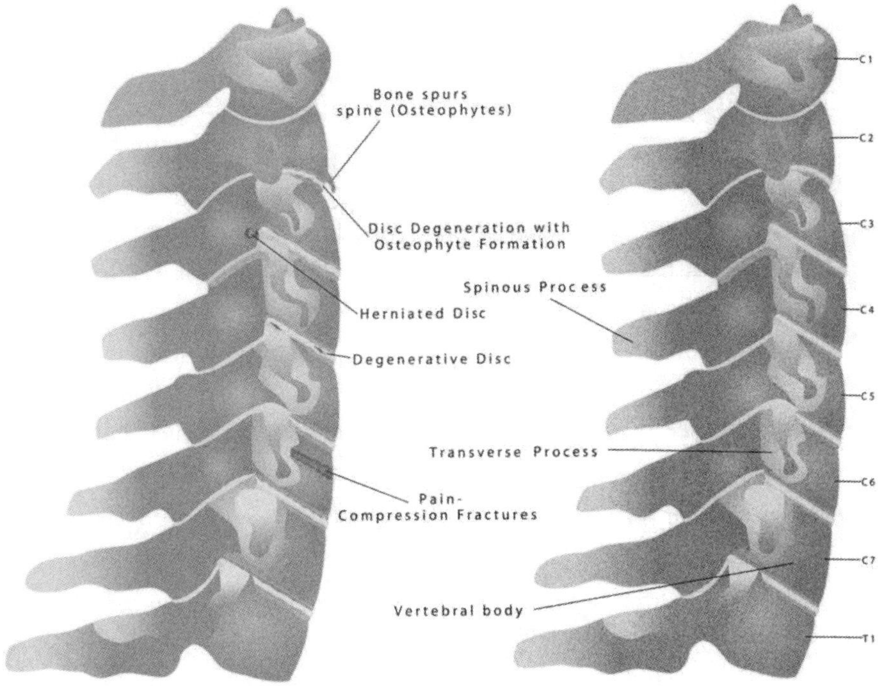

SPINE ANATOMY CERVICAL REGION

Neck: Cervical Herniated Nucleus Prolapse (HNP)/Herniated Disc/Bulging Disc/Spondylolisthesis

Herniated disc, bulging disc, slipped disc, herniated nucleus pulposus (HNP)- Spinal discs are soft, compressible discs that separate **interlocking bones** (vertebrae) that make up the spine. These discs act as shock absorbers for the spine, allowing it to flex, bend, and twist. Bulging, herniated or ruptured discs can occur when the intervertebral discs become compressed and **bulge outward** (herniate) or **rupture,** causing nerve irritation.

The tough covering of a disc in the spine can **tear** (rupture), causing pain. The soft, jelly-like interior may **bulge out** (herniate) through the covering, causing more pain. Pain occurs because the bulge puts pressure on the spinal nerve root next to it. Sometimes the nerve is damaged. A disc may herniate because of a sudden injury or repeated minor injuries.

Where the pain occurs depends on which disc is herniated and which spinal nerve is affected. **The pain is felt along the pathway of the nerve compressed by the herniated disc**. The pain varies from slight to debilitating and movement intensifies the pain. Numbness and muscle weakness may also occur.

It is possible for cervical disc herniation (and all spinal disc herniation) to completely heal and fully resolve. In fact, there are published case reports of **acupuncture** promoting this self-healing **("Acupuncture and Spontaneous Regression of Radiculopathic Cervical Herniated Disc", *J Pharmacopuncture* 2012 Jun; 15(2): 36-39).**
https://www.ncbi.nlm.nih.gov/pmc/articles/PMC4331934/

Acupuncture helps many patients with disc problems to experience a reduction of their pain and resume normal work and lifestyle for years.

Patients with disc issues are occasionally told they need surgery. **Patients should always get a second opinion regarding any surgery, especially spinal surgery**. A 2013 study of spine surgery **second opinions** showed that of 183 second opinions seen over 20 months, the second opinion surgeon documented that the previous spine surgeon recommended an **"unnecessary" surgery 60.7%** of the time, the **"wrong" surgery 33.3%** of the time, and the **"right" surgery 6%** of the time **("Are Recommended Spine Operations Either Unnecessary or Too Complex? Evidence from Second Opinions", *Surg Neurol Int.,* 2013; 4 (Suppl5); S353-S358).**
https://www.ncbi.nlm.nih.gov/pmc/articles/PMC3841934/

Spondylolisthesis- Spondylolisthesis is the forward displacement of a vertebra over a lower vertebra. The forward slippage of the vertebra can lead to **spinal stenosis** and **radiculopathy** (radiating pain, numbness, and/or weakness along the path of the nerve), which results in muscles that are tight and painful in response to movement. Spondylolisthesis is classified according to severity, from a grade 1 (mild) to a grade 4 (severe).

Acupuncture has been shown to help many patients with Grade 1 and 2 spondylolisthesis and associated disc problems to experience a **reduction** of their **pain** and **muscle spasms** and resume normal work and lifestyle for years. Unfortunately, with Grade 3 or 4 spondylolisthesis, acupuncture can only provide limited relief.

Recommended Treatment Protocol: Physical Exam and twelve treatments (2x/week for 6 weeks) is considered one course of treatment. Multiple courses of treatment may be necessary.

Treatment Goals: Reduce the frequency, intensity, and duration of neck pain, promote functional improvement and quality of life.

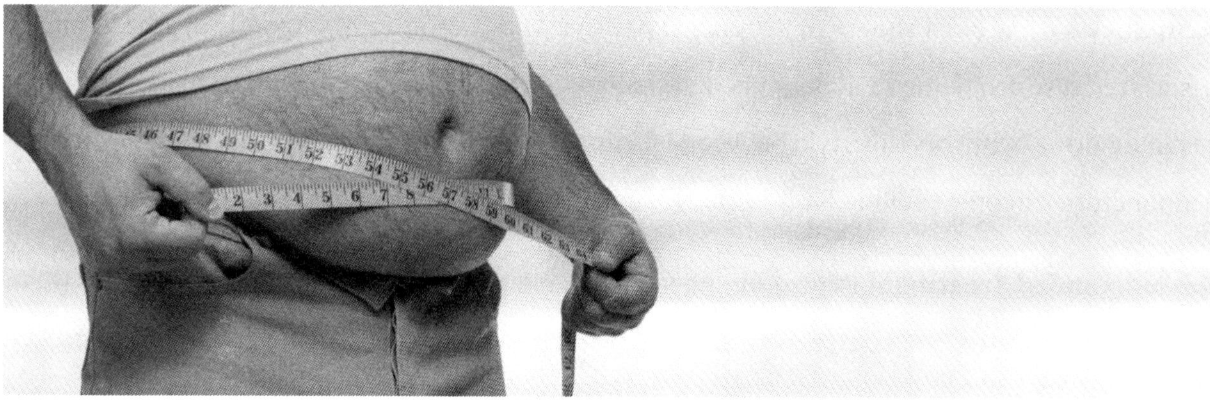

Obesity

Obesity means having too much body fat. It is different from being overweight, meaning one weighs too much. Technically, obesity is defined as having a **body mass index (BMI)** of **30** or greater. According to the **Centers for Disease Control (CDC)**, more than **one third (36.5%)** of U.S. adults have obesity.

Obesity increases the risks of **health problems**. Obesity-related conditions include heart disease, stroke, type 2 diabetes, and certain types of cancer. These conditions represent the **leading causes of death** in the United States.

The estimated **medical cost** of obesity in the U.S. was $147 billion in 2008, and the medical costs for people who have obesity are **significantly greater** than those of normal weight individuals. **https://www.cdc.gov/obesity/data/adult.html**

Because of these facts, if someone is obese, it should be an absolute priority to get to a normal weight and acupuncture can play a role in this process.

In a recent review and meta-analysis of published medical studies, acupuncture was shown to be able to reduce the **body mass index (BMI)** of obese patients, as well as **body fat mass (BFM)**, and **waist** and **hip circumference.** The authors concluded "Acupuncture appears to be an effective treatment for simple obesity" **("Acupuncture for the Treatment of Obesity in Adults: A Systematic Review and Meta-Analysis"** ***Post Grad Med J*** **2017 Jul 8).** **https://www.ncbi.nlm.nih.gov/pubmed/28689171**

Further, another study also evaluated the effects of electro-acupuncture on **visceral** and **hepatic fat** in women with **abdominal obesity,** and found that "Based on MRI evaluation, this randomized, controlled study proved that electro-acupuncture reduces **body mass index (BMI)** and **waist circumference**, as well as **visceral adipose tissue volume** and **hepatic fat fraction** in women with abdominal obesity **("Effect of Electro-Acupuncture on Visceral and Hepatic Fat in Women with Abdominal Obesity: A Randomized Controlled Study Based on Magnetic Resonance Imaging"** ***J Altern Complement Med 2017*** **Apr; 23(4): 285-294).** **https://www.ncbi.nlm.nih.gov/pubmed/28394670**

It is important to note that in this study, the patients received acupuncture three times per week for three months (**36 treatments**). This illustrates the importance of getting a sufficient number of treatments in order to achieve the full benefits of what acupuncture can do (for more info see **"How Frequently Should I Receive Acupuncture")**.

Recommended Treatment Protocol: Physical exam and 36 visits (3x/week for three months). Depending on goals, multiple courses of treatment may be necessary. **Lifestyle modification can significantly reduce the number of treatments needed.**

Treatment Goals: Reduction of body mass index.

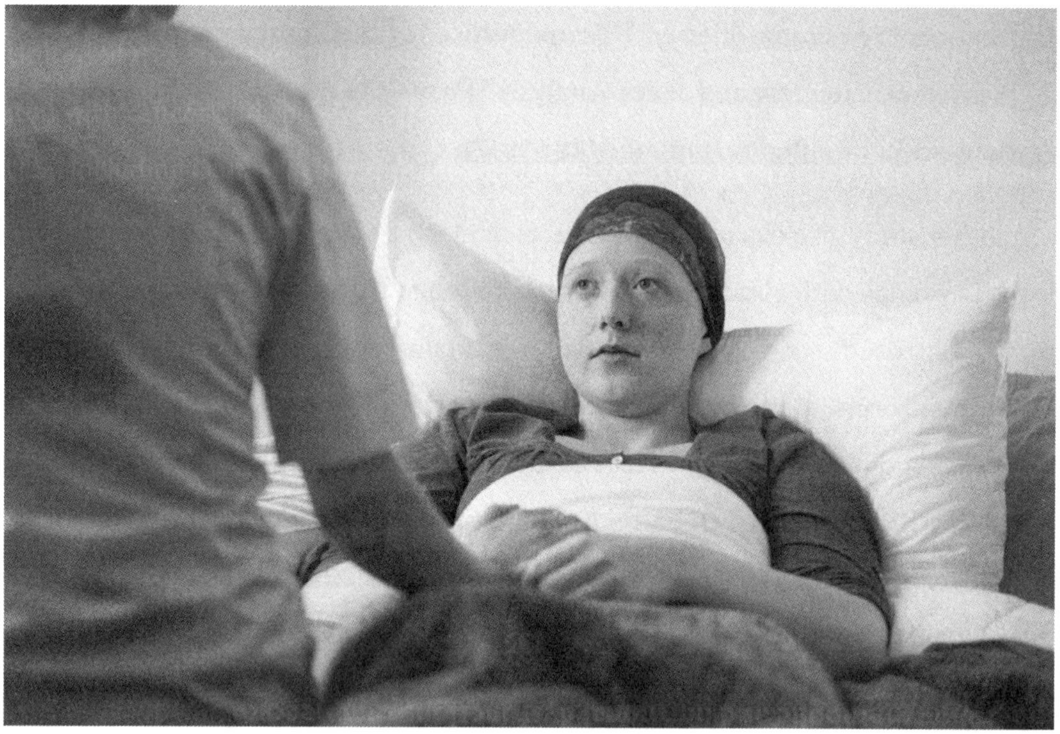

Oncology Support

Cancer is a group of diseases involving **abnormal cell growth** with the potential to spread to other parts of the body. There are over 100 different types of cancer and each is classified by the type of cell that is initially affected.

According to the **American Cancer Society**, cancer is the second most common cause of death in the U.S. In 2014 there were an estimated 14,738,719 living with cancer in America, and it's estimated that there will be over 1,500,000 new cases of cancer diagnoses every year. **https://www.cancer.gov/**

In the United States, **acupuncture** is used to treat a variety of **symptoms** and **conditions** associated with cancer and the **side effects** of cancer treatments. A number of cancer centers in the U.S., including **Dana-Farber Cancer Institute (DFCI) in Boston, Memorial Sloan-**

Kettering Cancer Center in New York, and **M.D. Anderson Cancer Center** in Houston are integrating acupuncture into modern oncology.

Randomized Clinical Trials (RCT's) have demonstrated that acupuncture is safe and effective for chemotherapy-induced nausea and vomiting. Research also suggests that acupuncture may be helpful in managing cancer related pain, post-operative pain, chemotherapy related neutropenia (low white blood cell count), cancer fatigue, radiation-induced xerostomia (dry mouth) and possibly insomnia, anxiety, and quality of life (*"The* Value of Acupuncture in Cancer Care", ***Hematol Oncol Clin North Am, 2008 August; 22(4):631).*** **https://www.ncbi.nlm.nih.gov/pmc/articles/PMC2642987/**

Breast Cancer, Hot Flashes: "Acupuncture in association with enhanced self-care is an effective integrative intervention for managing hot flashes and improving quality of life in women with breast cancer" **("Acupuncture as an Integrative Approach for the Treatment of Hot Flashes in Women with Breast Cancer: A Prospective Multicenter Randomized Controlled Trial",** ***J Clin Oncol,*** **2016 May 20; 34(15): 1795-802). https://www.ncbi.nlm.nih.gov/pubmed/27022113**

Breast Cancer, Joint Pain: "Women with **aromatase inhibitor** associated joint pain treated with acupuncture had significant improvement of joint pain and stiffness which was not seen with sham acupuncture. Acupuncture is an effective and well-tolerated strategy for managing this common treatment-related side effect" **("Randomized, Blinded, Sham-Controlled Trial of Acupuncture for the Management of Aromatase Inhibitor-Associated Joint Symptoms in Women with early-Stage Breast Cancer",** ***Journal of Clinical Oncology,*** **V28, No.7, March 1, 2010). https://www.ncbi.nlm.nih.gov/pubmed/20100963**

Chemotherapy: "Applying acupuncture at particular acupoints can influence tissue distribution of **Paclitaxel** (chemotherapy drug). Acupuncture resulted in an obvious **decrease** of Paclitaxel distribution in the **kidney** and delayed distribution in the **liver**. Meanwhile, it increased the time of metabolism. Acupuncture at BL13 (major acupoint for the lung) facilitated the delivery of Paclitaxel to the lung more effectively than did acupuncture at DU10 (an acupoint located in the same region)" **("Effects of Acupuncture on the Tissue Distribution of Paclitaxel in Lung**

Carcinoma Mice", *Chin L Integr Med,* 2014 Jun 13).
https://link.springer.com/article/10.1007/s11655-014-1819-1

Chemotherapy: At least one study has shown that adding **vitamin B-12** (in the form of methylcobalamin) with acupuncture yields the best results for chemotherapy-induced peripheral neuropathy **("Acupuncture Combined with Methylcobalamin for the Treatment of Chemotherapy-Induced Peripheral Neuropathy in Patient with Multiple Myeloma", *BMC Cancer,* 2017; 17:40). https://www.ncbi.nlm.nih.gov/pmc/articles/PMC5223334/**

Dry Mouth: "Acupuncture at LI2 was associated with **neuronal activations** absent during sham acupuncture stimulation. Neuroimaging signal changes appear correlated to **saliva production**" **("Functional Magnetic Resonance Imaging (fMRI) Changes and Saliva Production Associated with Acupuncture at LI-2 Acupuncture Point: A Randomized Controlled Study", *BMC Complement Altern Med,* 2008; 8:37).**
https://www.ncbi.nlm.nih.gov/pmc/articles/PMC2474572/

Lung Cancer: "Acupuncture may be an effective approach for improving **symptoms** (pain and well-being in particular) in lung cancer patients" **("The Potential Role for Acupuncture in Treating Symptoms in Patients with Lung Cancer: an Observational Longitudinal Study", *Current Oncology,* V20, No.3 June 2013).**
https://www.ncbi.nlm.nih.gov/pmc/articles/PMC3671020/

Chemotherapy Induced Nausea and Vomiting: "Acupuncture is **effective** in preventing chemotherapy induced **nausea** and **vomiting** and in promoting better quality of life with fewer adverse effects" **("Efficacy of Acupuncture in Prevention of Delayed Chemotherapy Induced Nausea and Vomiting in Gynecologic Cancer Patients", *Gynecol Oncol,* 2015 Jan; 136(1): 82-6). https://www.ncbi.nlm.nih.gov/pubmed/25449310/**

Post-Cancer Surgery Pain and Dry Mouth: "Significant **reductions** in **pain**, **dysfunction**, and **xerostomia** (dry mouth) were observed in patients receiving acupuncture versus usual care" **("Acupuncture for Pain and Dysfunction after Neck Dissection: Results of a Randomized Controlled Trial",** ***J Clin Oncol,*** **2010 May 20; 28(15): 2565-70). https://www.ncbi.nlm.nih.gov/pubmed/20406930**

Radiation-Induced Dry Mouth (that doesn't respond to medication): "Acupuncture using a standard protocol may contribute to less **xerostomia** (dry mouth) for some patients with **refractory symptoms** after radiotherapy" **("Acupuncture Technique for Pilocarpine-Resistant Xerostomia Following Radiotherapy for Head and Neck Malignancies",** ***Int J Radiation Oncology Biol Phys,*** **V50, No.2, pp353-357 2011). http://www.academia.edu/29701969/Acupuncture_for_pilocarpine-resistant_xerostomia_following_radiotherapy_for_head_and_neck_malignancies**

Dive Deeper into Biomedicine- Insights into Cancer Treatment

Modifying the **surface** of acupuncture needles in a **particular way** has shown some surprising benefits. In one study, acupuncture was given to lab rats with cancer every day for 40 weeks, using standard acupuncture needles in one group, and modified acupuncture needles in another group.

The results of the study are **very intriguing**. While **both groups** demonstrated a **reduction** in **tumor size**, the modified needle group was found to be **more effective** in reducing average tumor size, B-catenin expression levels, and number of aberrant crypt foci in the colon endothelium **("Enhanced Therapeutic Treatment of Colorectal Cancer Using Surface-Modified Nanoporous Acupuncture Needles",** ***Scientific Reports,*** **7, 12900, October 2017). https://www.nature.com/articles/s41598-017-11213-0**

Dive Deeper into Biomedicine- Insights into Cancer Treatment Con't.

In addition, there are other things besides drugs that oncology patients can do to reduce the risk of cancer recurrence, but once again, the information is not getting to the patients. For example, one study showed "Tamoxifen can reduce the risk for breast cancer recurrence by about 40%, whereas **physical activity** at a level of 9 **metabolic equivalents of task (METS)** per week **reduces the risk for recurrence by 50%**. Although **patients** and **physicians** are aware of the benefit of tamoxifen, they are often **not aware** of the **major survival advantage** of physical activity" **("Complementary Therapies Can Boost Survival in Cancer Patients", March 20, 2015). https://www.medscape.com/viewarticle/841801**

Recommended Treatment Protocol: Physical Exam and twelve treatments (2x/week for 6 weeks) is considered one course of treatment. Multiple courses of treatment may be necessary. **Each clinical scenario is different, and the acupuncture protocol will be individualized to the exact medical presentation.**

Treatment Goals: Assist patient in completing their cancer treatment and to recover from the effects of their cancer treatment, reduce side effects, and improve quality of life.

STAGES OF OSTEOPOROSIS

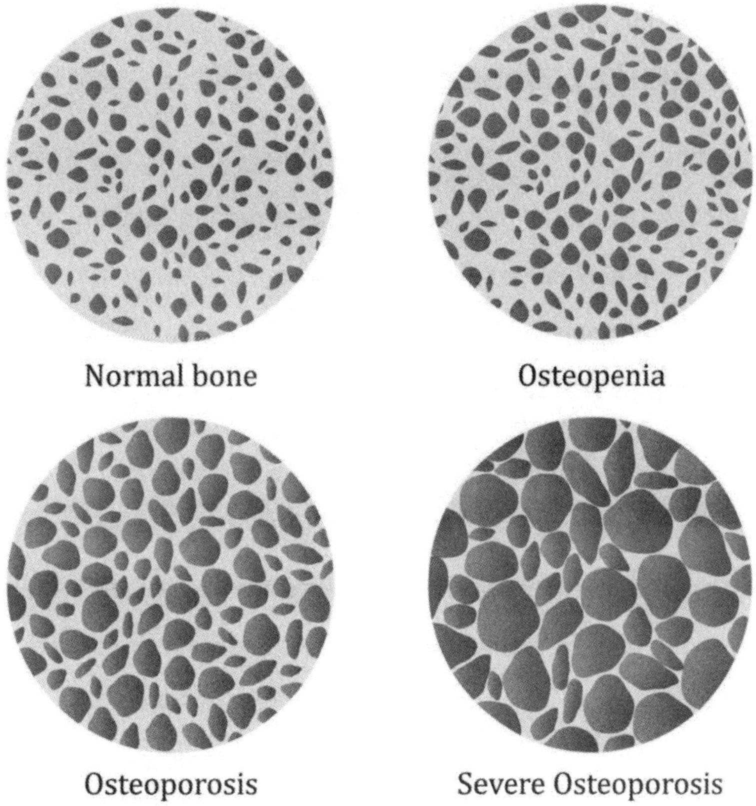

Osteoporosis/Osteopenia

Osteoporosis is a condition in which the **bones** become **weak** and **brittle**. **Osteopenia** is a condition in which the **bone mineral density** is **less** than **normal**. Many doctors feel that **osteopenia** is a **precurso**r to **osteoporosis**. It is estimated that **50%** of the women in the U.S. between the ages of 45 and 75 will be affected by osteoporosis to some degree, with 16% experiencing **serious bone deterioration** that could lead to **fractures** and **injuries**.

Osteoporosis is a **pathology** which is tied to **hormonal deficiency**, **acidity imbalance**, and other **metabolic issues**. **Those diagnosed with osteoporosis should understand that they have underlying metabolic and hormonal dysfunctions that need to be addressed.** Instead

patients are simply instructed to **"take calcium"** or prescribed a **bisphosphonate**, the value of which has been questioned in recent years.
http://www.ti.ubc.ca/2011/02/23/bisphosphonates-do-they-prevent-or-cause-bone-fractures/

Traditionally, **acupuncture** was used to keep people **strong** and **healthy** even into advanced age. Both the **Emperor** and **martial arts masters** dating back to the famous **Shaolin Temple** used acupuncture and Traditional Chinese Medicine (TCM) herbal formulas to increase their **bone density** and help **repair fractures** sustained in combat if they should occur.

Modern researchers are just starting to look at the role **acupuncture** can play in the **prevention** and treatment of osteopenia and osteoporosis. In one animal study, scientists first gave rats osteopenia, then gave them 16 weeks of acupuncture. At the conclusion of the study, it was determined that the **weight** and **structure** of the acupuncture-treated rats had **improved** compared to the control group. Researchers stated "Our findings show that acupuncture may prevent osteopenia" **("Preventative and Therapeutic Effects of Acupuncture on Bone Mass in Osteopenic Ovariectomized Rats"** ***Am J Chin Med*** **2004 32(3): 427-43). https://www.ncbi.nlm.nih.gov/pubmed/15344426**

Another animal study had similar results, showing that two specific acupoints appear to have **specific actions** on **bone**. The acupuncture-treated rats had **improvements** in the **strength**, **weight,** and **structure** of their **bones ("The More Efficacious Acupoints of** ***Zusanli*** **and** ***Sanyinjiao*** **than that of Non-Acupoints on Bone Mass in Osteopenic Ovariectomized Rats"** ***Chin J Integr Med*** **2005 Sept; 11(3): 209-16).**
https://www.ncbi.nlm.nih.gov/pubmed/16181537

Finally, several animal studies have shown that **electro-acupuncture** at specific points **improved bone** and made **positive biomechanical changes**:

"Effect of Electro-Acupuncture on ***Mingmen*** **(GV4) on Bone Morphogenetic Protein-2 Expression in Osteoporosis Rats"** ***Zhen Ci Yan Jiu*** **2014 Apr; 39(2):130-5.**
https://www.ncbi.nlm.nih.gov/pubmed/24818497

"Electro-Acupuncture Stimulation at CV4 Prevents Ovariectomy-Induced Osteoporosis in Rats Via Wnt-B-Catenin Signaling" ***Mol Med Rep*** **2016 Mar; 13(3): 2485-91. https://www.ncbi.nlm.nih.gov/pubmed/26846191**

It's important to note that in these animal studies, acupuncture was given every day for thirty days, with a one day break every ten days (thirty treatments over a thirty three day period). For more information on the importance of doing a high number of treatments over a short period of time, see **"How Frequently Should I Get Acupuncture?"**.

Traditional Chinese Medicine (TCM) herbal formulas have also been shown to increase bone density. In a recent study, researchers tested a compound derived from the TCM herb **"Dang Shen"** in human and mouse bone cells and a mouse model. They found it **prevented bone loss** and **increased** the **bone mineral density** of the mice treated by 35% without causing side effects. **("New Osteoporosis Treatment Uses Traditional Chinese Herb to Prevent Bone Loss",** ***Journal of Bone and Mineral Research,*** **University of British Columbia News, August 29, 2017). https://news.ubc.ca/2017/08/29/new-osteoporosis-treatment-uses-traditional-chinese-herb-to-prevent-bone-loss/**

Recommended Treatment Protocol: Physical exam and thirty treatments over a ten week period (3x/week for ten weeks) is considered one course of treatment. **Lifestyle modification including reducing alcohol intake, smoking cessation, adding weight bearing exercise, and optimized nutrition can dramatically reduce the number of acupuncture treatments needed.** Depending on lifestyle factors, secondary causes of osteoporosis, and degree of osteoporosis, multiple courses of treatment may be necessary.

Treatment Goals: Increase strength, weight, and density of bone mass, and increase biomechanical functionality, thereby reducing the risk of fractures and improving quality of life.

PARKINSON'S DISEASE

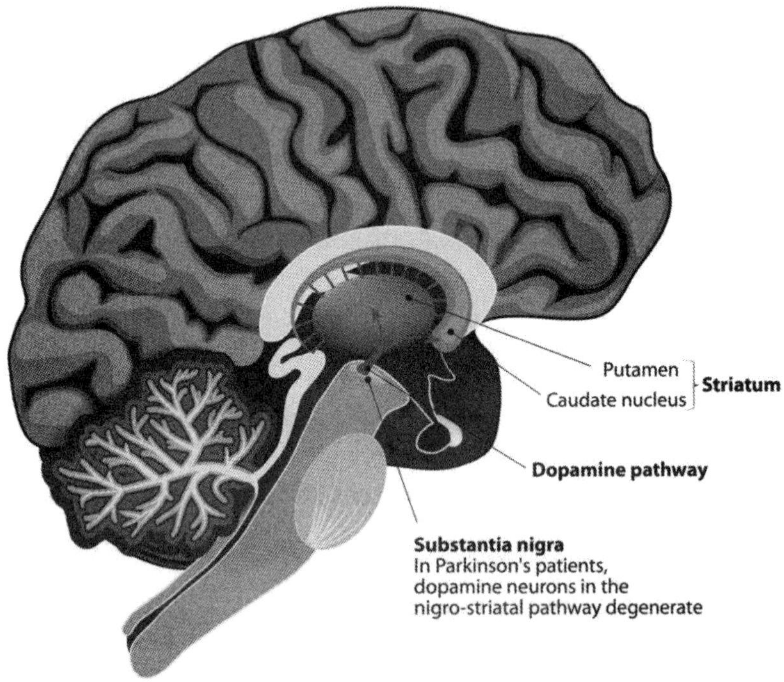

Parkinson's Disease

Parkinson's Disease (PD) is a progressive disorder of the **nervous system** that affects **movement.** It is caused by **nerve cell damage** in the **brain** that causes **dopamine levels** to drop. **Dopamine** is a **neurotransmitter** that helps to **regulate movement** and **emotional** responses. PD affects more than 200,000 people in the United States.

The cause of Parkinson's disease is **unknown** but both **genetic** and **environmental triggers** appear to play a role. People with Parkinson's have **low brain dopamine** concentrations. Unfortunately, dopamine can't be given directly because it can't enter the brain. Presently there is no cure but medications are currently prescribed to help with walking, tremor, and movement.

Statins are a class of drugs commonly used to lower cholesterol. The use of statins has been called into question in recent years, and there is some evidence that their use is linked to Parkinson's Disease **("Statin Use Linked to Increased Parkinson's Risk" (American Neurological Association (ANA) 2016 Annual Meeting). http://www.medscape.com/viewarticle/870996**

Animal studies have shown that **electro-acupuncture** stimulates a **neural circuit** that results in the release of dopamine **(Regulating Innate Immunity with Dopamine and Electro-Acupuncture"** ***Nature Medicine*** **20, 239-241,2014). http://www.nature.com/nm/journal/v20/n3/full/nm.3501.html?foxtrotcallback=true**

Animal studies also show **electro-acupuncture** enhances the **synaptic dopamine availability** to **improve motor function ("Acupuncture Enhances the Synaptic Dopamine Availability to Improve Motor Function in a Mouse Model of Parkinson's Disease",** ***PLos One*** **2011; 6(11):e27566). https://www.ncbi.nlm.nih.gov/pubmed/22132113**

A thorough review of all current research on acupuncture for PD (clinical studies, animal studies, and functional MRI imaging studies) was completed in 2015. After analyzing the data, the researchers concluded:

"First, **acupuncture** is **anti-inflammatory**, **anti-oxidative**, **anti-apoptotic** (prevents cell death), **neurotrophic** (helps repair nerves), and **increases dopamine availability**, **restores post-synaptic changes due to dopamine loss** (repairs damage caused by low dopamine) and **changes** certain **gene** and **protein expressions**".

"Second, **acupuncture re-activates** the **dysfunctional brain circuitry** for motor and non-motor function and relieves the symptoms. Clinical trials suggest that acupuncture is effective in non-motor symptoms in sleep, rest, and depression".

"Another clear benefit is that **acupuncture** can **reduce** the **medication** (therapeutic L-dopa) treatment dose and therefore **lower** the **risk** of its related **side effects** (L-dopa induced dyskinesia)".

"**Acupuncture**, as a potential **neuroprotective agent**, is supported by preclinical animal studies with consistent efficacy and pilot **clinical trials** show **positive evidence** of acupunctures benefit in treating PD, and it is **safe** and **well tolerated**" **("Acupuncture for Parkinson's Disease: A Review of Clinical, Animal, and Functional Magnetic Resonance Imaging Studies",** ***J Tradit Chin Med 2015*** **Dec 15; 35(6): 709-717).**
http://www.sciencedirect.com/science/article/pii/S0254627215301643

Finally, a recent animal study showed that **electro-acupuncture** produces **sustained motor improvement** for at least **four weeks after treatment** in mice with Parkinson's disease **("Electro-Acupuncture Produces the Sustained Motor Improvement in 6-Hydroxydopamine-Lesioned Mice",** ***PLos One*** **2016 Feb 19; 11(2): e0149111).**
https://www.ncbi.nlm.nih.gov/pubmed/26894437

Dive Deeper into Biomedicine- Insights into Parkinson's Disease

Although the **cause** of **Parkinson's Disease (PD)** is **unknown**, researchers have known for some time that too much **iron buildup** in the brain is associated with PD, as well as other neurodegenerative diseases **("Too Much Iron in the Brain May Lead to Parkinson's Disease, May Damage Neurons",** ***Medical Daily*****, Jan 25, 2016).** **http://www.medicaldaily.com/parkinsons-disease-excess-iron-370884**

Further, researchers have focuses on **iron concentrations** in a particular area of the brain, the **"substantia nigra"**,which is the area in which the **neurons** that **produce dopamine** are concentrated **("Nigral Iron Elevation is an Invariable Feature of Parkinson's Disease and is a Sufficient Cause of Neurodegeneration",** ***Biomed Res Int.*** **2014; 2014: 581256).** **https://www.ncbi.nlm.nih.gov/pubmed/24527451**

Animal studies have shown that **acupuncture** may **inhibit iron-related oxidative damage** in the substantia nigra and may **prevent** the **deleterious alteration** of **iron metabolism** in mice with Parkinson's **("Acupuncture Inhibits Ferric Iron Deposition and Ferritin-Heavy Chain Reduction in an MPTP-Induced Parkinsonism Model",** ***Neurosci Lett.*** **2009 Jan 30; 450(2): 92-6). https://www.ncbi.nlm.nih.gov/pubmed/19056464**

Often times, acupuncture research leads to breakthroughs in ways the researchers hadn't expected. Acupuncture research into PD has helped give insight into this complex disorder. In a 2013 study, not only did acupuncture provide clear positive effects, but information was obtained which showed how the disease manifests.

The researchers stated "We showed that **acupuncture stimulation** in Parkinson's models had generated valuable **mechanistic insight** of Parkinson's and showed that **acupuncture treatment** is in fact a **neuroprotective therapy** that **increases** the release of various **neuroprotective agents** such as brain-derived neurotrophic factor, glial cell line-derived neurotrophic factor, and cyclophilin A".

"In addition, **acupuncture** therapy **slows cell death process** and attenuates **oxidative stress** to **dopaminergic neurons** in the substantia nigra".

Dive Deeper into Biomedicine- Insights into Parkinson's Disease Con't.

"Further, acupuncture therapy **modulates neuronal activity** of the **basal ganglia** output structures" **("Current Development of Acupuncture Research in Parkinson's Disease",** ***Int Rev Neurobiol,*** **2013; 111: 141-58). https://www.ncbi.nlm.nih.gov/pubmed/24215921**

Other interesting studies showing a **positive effect** of acupuncture on Parkinson's Disease include:

"Acupuncture Inhibits Microglial Activation and Inflammatory Events in the MPTP-Induced Mouse Model", ***Brain Res*** **2007 Feb 2; 1131(1): 211-9. https://www.ncbi.nlm.nih.gov/pubmed/17173870**

"Acupuncture Stimulation on GB34 Activates Neural Responses Associated with Parkinson's Disease", ***CNS Neurosci Ther,*** **2012 Sep; 18(9): 781-90. https://www.ncbi.nlm.nih.gov/pubmed/22943145**

"Acupuncture on GB34 Activates the Precentral Gyrus and Prefrontal Cortex in Parkinson's Disease" ***BMJ Complement and Altern Med*** **2014, 14:336. https://www.ncbi.nlm.nih.gov/pubmed/25220656**

Recommended Treatment Protocol: Physical Exam and twelve treatments (2x/week for 6 weeks) is considered one course of treatment. Multiple courses of treatment may be necessary. Maintenance treatments will be necessary.

Treatment Goals: Enhance synaptic dopamine availability to improve motor function, reduce medication dosage needed therefore reduce risk of L-dopa induced dyskinesia, improve physiological homeostasis to reduce associated symptoms.

PERIPHERAL NEUROPATHY

NERVE DAMAGE

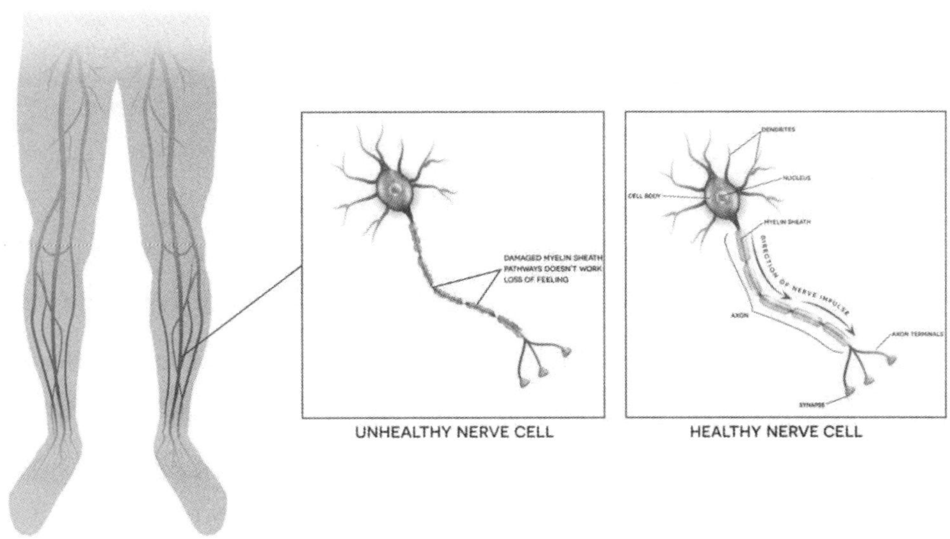

Peripheral Neuropathy

Peripheral Neuropathy (PN) is a result of damage to your **peripheral nerves.** It often causes **weakness, numbness**, and **pain**, usually in the hands and feet. It can also affect other areas of your body.

There are over 100 types of **peripheral neuropathies** and therefore **many possible causes**. Clinically, the most common causes are **nerve damage** from **trauma** or **repetitive stress**, **metabolic** and **endocrine disorders**, **toxicity**, **nutritional deficiency**, and **genetic disorders**.

Physical injury (trauma and repetitive stress) is the most **common cause** of acquired neuropathy. **Peripheral nerves** have the ability to **regenerate axons** (as long as the nerve cell itself has not died) which may lead to **functional recovery** with **treatment** over time.

Recent studies demonstrate that "acupuncture significantly improves **motor nerve conduction velocity** and **amplitude** and also **promotes functional nerve repair**" ***(Neural Regeneration Research V10, no.1 (2015):128)*** **and "acupuncture improves nerve conduction in peripheral neuropathy"** ***(Eur J Neurol*** **2007 Mar; 14(3): 276-81*).***
https://www.ncbi.nlm.nih.gov/pubmed/17355547

Diabetic Peripheral Neuropathy

A recent study of 2,000 young diabetes patients showed that 7% of those with type 1 diabetes and 20% of those with type 2 diabetes had **diabetic peripheral neuropathy (DPN)**. And these are **young** diabetics. The same study showed **"alarming rates"** of increase in DPN for **every 5 years** that people have diabetes **(*Diabetes Care*, July 2017)**.
http://care.diabetesjournals.org/content/early/2017/06/30/dc17-0179

In DPN the blood glucose must be adequately regulated. Strict control of blood glucose levels has been shown to reduce neuropathic symptoms and avoid further nerve damage. In addition, regulating blood glucose levels can reduce need for oral insulin such as Metformin, and Metformin has been correlated with vitamin B-12 deficiency which can also cause neuropathy (see **"Nutritional Deficiencies"** below).

Diabetic Peripheral Neuropathy is **twice** as **common** in **smokers** than in nonsmokers. Smoking constricts blood vessels that supply nutrients to peripheral nerves and can worsen neuropathic symptoms and slow the repair of damaged tissue (see **"Stop Smoking"** for more information).

Acupuncture has been shown to relieve diabetic peripheral neuropathy **("Fifteen-Day Acupuncture Treatment Relieves Diabetic Peripheral Neuropathy", *Journal of Acupuncture and Meridian Studies*, V3, Issue 2, June 2010, pp95-103).**
http://www.sciencedirect.com/science/article/pii/S2005290110600180

Other Causes of Peripheral Neuropathy

Exposure to Toxins- Exposure to toxins may **damage nerves** and cause peripheral neuropathy. Common causes include **medication toxicity** (either intentional, as in chemotherapy, or unintentional as in an unwanted side effect of medication to treat another condition),

environmental or industrial toxins (lead, mercury, arsenic, insecticides, solvents), and **heavy alcohol consumption**. When neuropathy is caused by toxic exposure, the most important step is to **discontinue the exposure**. If that is not possible, as in chemotherapy, then acupuncture must be initiated as soon as possible.

At least one study has shown that adding **vitamin B-12** (in the form of methylcobalamin) with acupuncture yields the best results for chemotherapy induced peripheral neuropathy **("Acupuncture Combined with Methylcobalamin for the Treatment of Chemotherapy-Induced Peripheral Neuropathy in Patient with Multiple Myeloma",** ***BMC Cancer,*** **2017; 17:40). https://www.ncbi.nlm.nih.gov/pmc/articles/PMC5223334/**

Nutritional Deficiencies- Nutritional deficiencies are very common today. **Vitamin B-12** deficiency can cause nerve damage and neuropathy even when no anemia develops. There are many causes of vitamin B-12 deficiency. Older people may have a B-12 deficiency because stomach acidity is low, reducing the absorption of B-12 from food. Abnormal growth of bacteria in the small intestine may reduce the absorption as well.

Also, 50% of patients who have had **gastric bypass surgery** have nutritional deficiencies, including vitamin B-12 deficiency **("Nutritional Deficiencies after Gastric Bypass Surgery",** ***The Journal of the American Osteopathic Association*** **Nov. 2009 Vol. 109 601-604). http://jaoa.org/article.aspx?articleid=2093757 .**

Medications- Medications can interfere with B-12 absorption. In fact, **10%-30%** of patients who take the diabetes drug Metformin have vitamin B-12 deficiency **("Association of Vitamin B-12 Deficiency and Metformin Use in Patients with Type 2 Diabetes",** ***J Korean Med Sci*** **2014 Jul 29 (7):965-972). https://www.ncbi.nlm.nih.gov/pmc/articles/PMC4101785/**

Further, people who take **proton pump inhibitors (PPI's)** for acid reflux have a 65% greater chance of B-12 deficiency **(Mayo Clinic)**.

> Vitamin B-12 deficiency can be adequately addressed with the administration of B-12 via intramuscular injection. This is crucial because nerve damage from B-12 deficiency can become permanent if not treated.

Dive Deeper into Biomedicine-Medical Management of Peripheral Neuropathy

The **medical** protocol for PN, like the **acupuncture** protocol, is based on the cause of the neuropathy. If neuropathy is caused by a **medical condition,** that condition will be addressed medically. Mild pain is managed with anti-inflammatory drugs (NSAIDs). When this is not enough, other medications may be prescribed including several classes of drugs: antidepressants, anticonvulsants, antiarrythmics, narcotics, and topical analgesics. It is **important** to note that **all drugs** have a risk of **side effects**, including cumulative **drug toxicity.**

When medications do not provide adequate relief, **surgical interventions** may be used. Some surgical procedures reduce pain by **destroying nerves.** This approach is appropriate only for pain caused by a single nerve and when other forms of treatment have failed to provide relief. Peripheral neuropathies that involve more diffuse nerve damage, such as diabetic neuropathies, are **not** amenable to surgical intervention **(Peripheral Neuropathy Fact Sheet, National Institute of Neurological Disorders and Stroke). www.ninds.nih.gov**

Recommended Treatment Protocol: Physical Exam (including blood work) and twelve acupuncture treatments (2x/week for 6 weeks) is considered one course of treatment. Multiple courses of treatment may be necessary. **Maintenance treatment will be necessary**. However, each clinical scenario is different, and the treatment protocol will be individualized to the exact medical presentation. Depending on the cause of the neuropathy, additional treatment (herbal foot soaks, vitamin B-12 injections, smoking cessation, blood glucose regulation, etc.) may be indicated.

Treatment Goals: Reduce intensity, frequency, and/or duration of pain, repair damaged nerves.

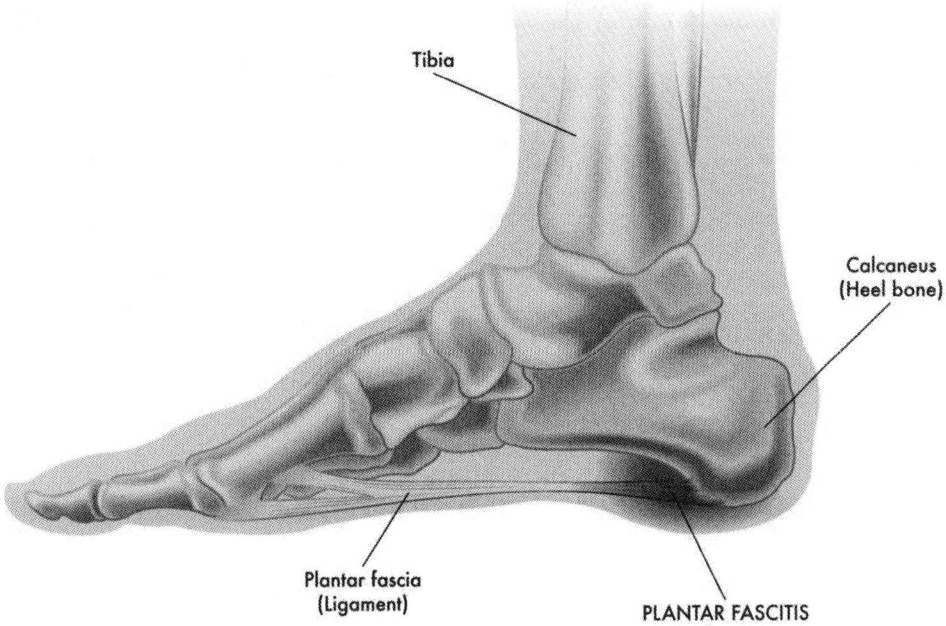

Plantar Fasciitis

Plantar Fasciitis (PF) is inflammation of the thick band of tissue that connects the heel bone to the toes. PF typically causes stabbing pain that is worse with the first steps in the morning. The exact cause of PF is **unknown,** but things which increase the **risk** of getting it are: **age**, **obesity**, performing certain types of **exercises** (running, jumping, dancing), **poor foot mechanics**, and **occupations** which keep you **standing** on your feet for long periods of time **(Mayo Clinic)**.

Acupuncture can be used to treat PF. In a 2012 study, patients received electro-acupuncture twice per week for five weeks (ten treatments total), along with **conventional care** (stretching exercises, shoe modification, and rescue pain killers). This group was compared to a control group, who only received conventional care.

Electro-acupuncture combined with conventional treatments provided a **success rate of 80%** in chronic plantar fasciitis, and the combination was more effective than conventional treatments alone. These effects lasted for at least **six weeks** after treatment **("Efficacy of Electro-Acupuncture in Chronic Plantar Fasciitis: A Randomized Controlled Trial" Am J Chin Med 2012; 40(6): 1167-76). https://www.ncbi.nlm.nih.gov/pubmed/23227789/**

A recent review of all the published medical literature found that acupuncture significantly reduced pain levels in patients with PF, but **these benefits were typically not seen until between four and eight weeks of treatment** **("How Effective is Acupuncture for Reducing Pain Due to Plantar Fasciitis?", *Singapore Med J* 2017; 58(2): 92-97). https://www.ncbi.nlm.nih.gov/pmc/articles/PMC5311890/**

However, in one interesting study, a **single acupuncture point** in the wrist (PC7) or hand (LI4) was used to treat PF. After treatment five times per week for two weeks **(10 treatments)**, acupuncture provided **significant** pain relief (**40% reduction** in **pain** at the **one month** follow up), and the results not only lasted for **six months** after treatment, they **continued to improve** over the **six months** after treatment **("Acupuncture Treatment for Plantar Fasciitis: A Randomized Controlled Trial with Six Months Follow Up" *Evid Based Complement and Altern Med 2011*; 2011: 154108). https://www.ncbi.nlm.nih.gov/pmc/articles/PMC3094706/**

Recommended Treatment Plan: Physical exam and 10 treatments (2x/week for five weeks) is considered one course of treatment. Multiple courses of treatment may be necessary.

Treatment Goal: Reduce the intensity, frequency, and/or duration of pain, prevent further complications including back, hip, or knee pain.

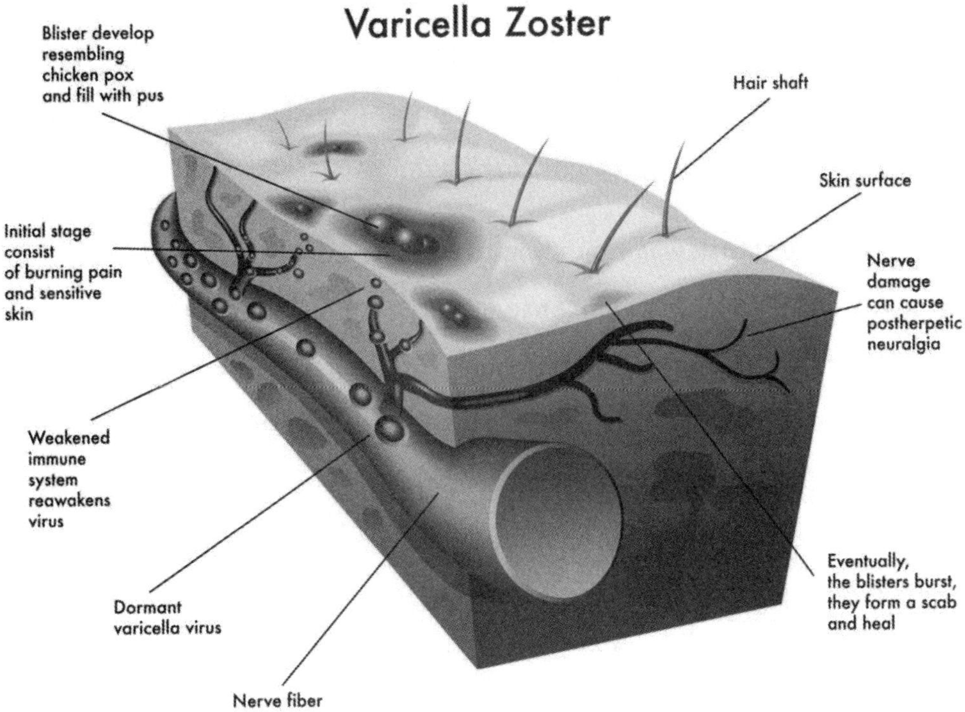

Shingles Pain

Herpes zoster, also known as **zoster** and **shingles,** is caused by the reactivation of the **varicella-zoster virus,** the same virus that causes **varicella** (chickenpox). Shingles is caused by a re-emergence of the virus, which has been lying dormant for years within the nerve cells. The virus causes **inflammation** of the **spinal ganglion** and a **vesicular eruption** along the area of distribution of the **affected spinal nerves**. Patients feel **excruciating, burning pain** or **tingling** in the affected area.

The **reactivation of the virus** may be **triggered** by trauma, diseases like pneumonia, injection of certain drugs, or prolonged stress which suppresses the immune function.

A **significant proportion** (18%-41%) of patients suffering with shingles experience intense or very intense pain. Frequently, these patients, despite the administration of **complex drug combinations**, cannot achieve pain control. They suffer with the **metabolic effects** and **side effects** of these drugs, but are still in **significant pain**.

In a recent study, **acupuncture** was compared to **standard drug therapy** from shingles pain. Researchers concluded "Patients with **intense** or **very intense pain** showed a **significant** and similar degree of pain relief using acupuncture and standard pharmacological therapy. Given that patients treated with **acupuncture carry** a **lower risk** of **cumulative drug toxicity**, acupuncture might be appropriately considered among the available therapeutic options for the control of severe acute HZ related pain" **("Acupuncture for the Treatment of Severe Acute Pain in Herpes Zoster: Results of a Nested, Open-Label Randomized Trial in the VZV Pain Study",** ***BMC Complement Altern Med*** **2011; 11:46).**
https://www.ncbi.nlm.nih.gov/pmc/articles/PMC3125389/

> Acupuncture can reduce pain levels, improve the pain-killing ability of opioid drugs (so the patient gets a greater benefit from a lower dosage), and speed healing and recovery from shingles.

Acupuncture **accelerates** the **healing process** through several mechanisms. Needling induces the release of **endorphins** which **reduces** the **stress level**. This process helps restore the function of the **immune system**, which in turn **deactivates** the **virus** and brings it under control. Local needling along the infected nerve stimulates an **anti-inflammatory** reaction and helps **recovery** or **regeneration of** the **damaged nerve fibers**.

Dive Deeper into Biomedicine-Insights into How Acupuncture Helps Shingles Pain

Acupuncture has been shown to **promote** functional nerve repair **("Improvement in Acupoint Selection for Acupuncture of Nerves Surrounding the Injury Site: Electro-Acupuncture with Governor Vessel with Local Meridian Acupoints",** ***Neural Regeneration Research*** **V10, no. 1 (2015): 128).**
https://www.ncbi.nlm.nih.gov/pmc/articles/PMC4357096/

Acupuncture has also been shown to assist the **immune system** in **self-regulating**. It is known that stress and anxiety disrupt the immune system. In an interesting study, acupuncture **normalized** the **biomarkers** of a reduced immune system in women with anxiety.

This same study showed that the most favorable effects of acupuncture on the immune functions appear **72 hours** after the acupuncture session and persist for **one month** after the end of the complete course of treatment **("Effect of Acupuncture Treatment on the Immune Function Impairment Found in Anxious Women",** ***Am J Chin Med*** **2007; 35(1):35-51).**
https://www.ncbi.nlm.nih.gov/pubmed/17265549

Recommended Treatment Protocol: Physical Exam and eight treatments (2x/week for 4 weeks) is considered one course of treatment. Multiple courses may be necessary.

Treatment Goals: Reduce the intensity, frequency, and/or duration of pain, reduce inflammation, strengthen immune system, regenerate damaged nerves, and calm stress.

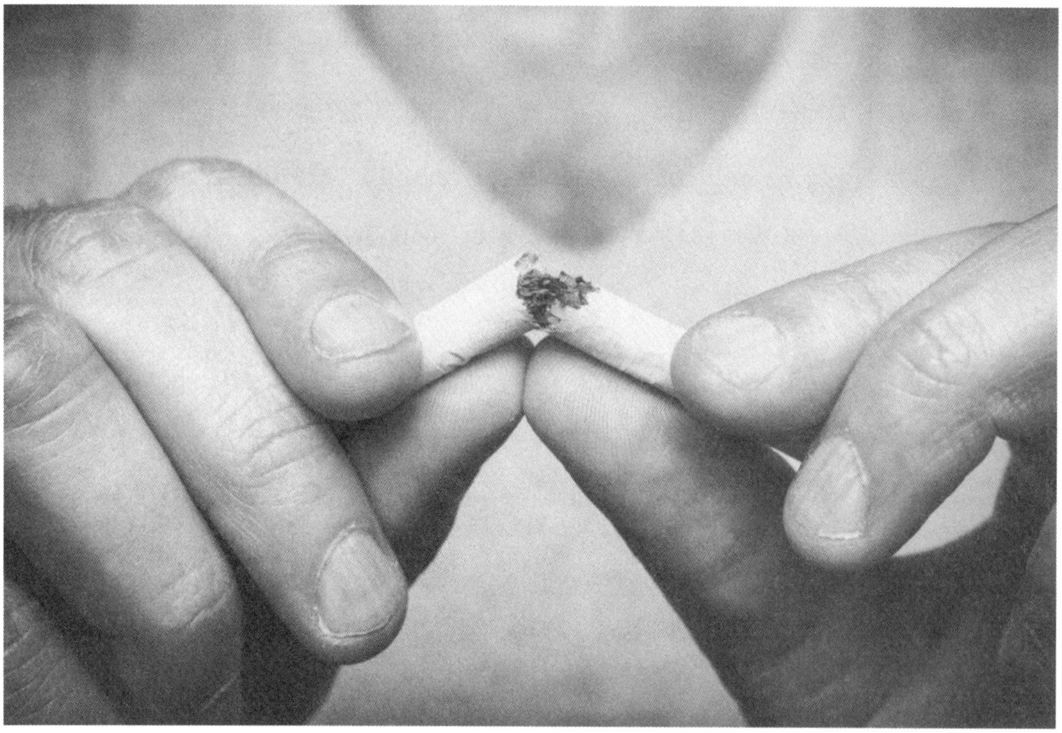

Stop Smoking

A large volume of data has accumulated on the issues of tobacco and health worldwide. **Cancer, cardiovascular diseases,** and **chronic obstructive pulmonary disease (COPD)** continue to be the main **health problems** associated with **smoking.** Because of the negative health effects and large number of people smoking, tobacco use is a **major public health problem** (which includes secondhand smoke exposure). **According to the CDC, 16 million Americans are living with a disease caused by smoking. Continued efforts to control and eliminate this addiction are a medical necessity.**

Yet in spite of the well-established health risks, approximately 47 million people smoke cigarettes in the U.S., and smoking prevalence is estimated at 28% of all men and 23% of all women nation-wide **("Cigarette Smoke and Adverse Health Effects: An Overview of Research Trends and Future Needs",** ***Int J Angio*****l. V16, No.3 Autumn 2007).**
https://www.ncbi.nlm.nih.gov/pmc/articles/PMC2733016/

It can be very difficult to quit smoking due to physical addiction, psychological addiction, triggers, stress, routine, social pressures, etc. However, acupuncture has been shown to assist in becoming smoke free and maintaining it for at least five years.

Acupuncture helps to **calm** and **relax** the **mind**, **reduce anxiety**, and alleviate **depression**. Specific acupuncture points on the ear and wrist are frequently used. Additional points are often added to help **suppress** the **appetite**, stimulate **repair** and **healing** of **organ systems**, and **reduce cravings**.

An interesting 2001 study on **smoking cessation** (quitting smoking) compared "true acupuncture" versus "sham acupuncture" (fake acupuncture). In the study, it was noted that the true acupuncture group had and maintained a **reduction** in smoking. The researchers concluded: "Adequate acupuncture treatment may help motivated smokers to **reduce** their smoking, or even **quit smoking** completely, and the effect may last for at least **5 years**. Acupuncture may affect the subjects' smoking by reducing their taste for tobacco and their desire to smoke. Different acupoints have been shown to have different effects on smoking cessation" **("Effect of Acupuncture on Smoking Cessation or Reduction: an 8-Month and 5-Year Follow-Up", *Prev Med.* 2001 Nov; 33(5): 364-72). https://www.ncbi.nlm.nih.gov/pubmed/11676576**

Other studies have had similar outcomes:

"Smoking Cessation after Acupuncture Treatment", *Int J Neurosci.* 2007 May; 117(5): 571-8. https://www.ncbi.nlm.nih.gov/pubmed/17464775

"Effects of Acupuncture on Smoking Cessation or Reduction for Motivated Smokers", *Prev Med.* 1997 Mar-Apr; 26(2): 208-14. https://www.ncbi.nlm.nih.gov/pubmed/9085389

Dive Deeper into Biomedicine- Negative Health Effects of Smoking

Besides the established associations of **smoking** to **cancer, cardiovascular disease**, and **COPD,** there are other **health risks** associated that are not as well-known but may have far reaching effects:

Vitamin B12 is a water soluble vitamin that plays an important role in the functioning of the brain and nervous system. Symptoms of **vitamin B12 deficiency** are many, but can include a reduced ability to think, irritability, depression, inflammation, poor muscle function, and decreased fertility.

The habit of smoking has been shown to reduce levels of vitamin B12 in the body **("Relationship of Tobacco Smoking with Serum Vitamin B12, Folic Acid, and Hematological Indices in Healthy Adults",** ***Public Health Nutri.*** **2003 Oct; 6(7): 675-81). https://www.ncbi.nlm.nih.gov/pubmed/14552668**

Adult smokers are **three times** as likely as non-smokers to have **periodontal disease ("Cigarette Smoking and the Periodontal Patient",** ***J Periodontal*** **2004 Feb; 75(2): 196-209). https://www.ncbi.nlm.nih.gov/pubmed/15068107**

Smoking increases the risk for **ALS ("Smoking and Risk for Amyptrophic Lateral Sclerosis: Analysis of the EPIC Cohort",** ***Ann Neurol 2009*** **Apr; 65(4): 378-85) https://www.ncbi.nlm.nih.gov/pubmed/19399866**

According to the **National Institute of Arthritis and Musculoskeletal and Skin Diseases**, smoking is a known risk factor for **osteoporosis https://www.bones.nih.gov/health-info/bone/osteoporosis/conditions-behaviors/bone-smoking**

Smoking is an environmental risk factor that can trigger **rheumatoid arthritis** in people with certain genes. **(www.arthritis.org)**

Dive Deeper into Biomedicine- Negative Health Effects of Smoking Con't.

Fathers who smoke **damage** their **DNA** and the effects are **passed down** to their **children** **("Cigarette Smoke Damages DNA in the Reproductive Cells of Fathers and these Changes are Inherited by the Offspring" (*Medical News Today*, June 26, 2012).** **https://www.medicalnewstoday.com/releases/246986.php**

Smoking increases the risk of **squamous cell carcinoma** by **52% ("Smoking Linked to Skin Cancer Risk", Medical News Today, June 23, 2012).** **https://www.medicalnewstoday.com/articles/246963.php**

Smoking is linked to **male dementia ("Smoking Speeds Up Male Cognitive Decline", Medical News Today, February 7, 2012). https://www.medicalnewstoday.com/articles/241241.php**

Smoking has been shown to promote the development of **lumbar herniation ("Is Smoking a Risk Factor for Lumbar Disc Herniation"?, *Eur Spine J* 2016 Jan; 25(1): 168-76).** **https://www.ncbi.nlm.nih.gov/pubmed/26160690**

According to the **Centers for Disease Control (CDC)**, smokers have **lower survival rates** after **surgery** and greater risk for **complications.** Smokers are also more likely to develop **peptic ulcers**, and smoking is linked to **erectile dysfunction**. **https://www.cdc.gov/tobacco/data_statistics/sgr/2004/highlights/other_effects/index.htm**

And finally, smokers are not only harming themselves, they are harming those around them. **Second hand** ("passive smoking") is associated with many medical conditions, including **type 2 diabetes** and **obesity ("Passive Smoking Tied to Type 2 Diabetes, Obesity", Catharine Paddock, PhD, Endocrine Society's 94th Annual Meeting).** **https://www.medicalnewstoday.com/articles/247110.php**

It is important to note that a pack-a-day smoker spends $2,250 per year just on cigarettes. When the costs of **healthcare,** lower **quality of life,** and **early death** are factored in, the costs are **exponentially higher**.

<u>Recommended Treatment Protocol:</u> Physical exam and eight treatments (2x/week for four weeks) is considered one course of treatment. Multiple courses of treatment may be necessary, and maintenance treatments may be necessary.

<u>Treatment Goal</u>: Reduce or eliminate tobacco use.

Types of Stroke

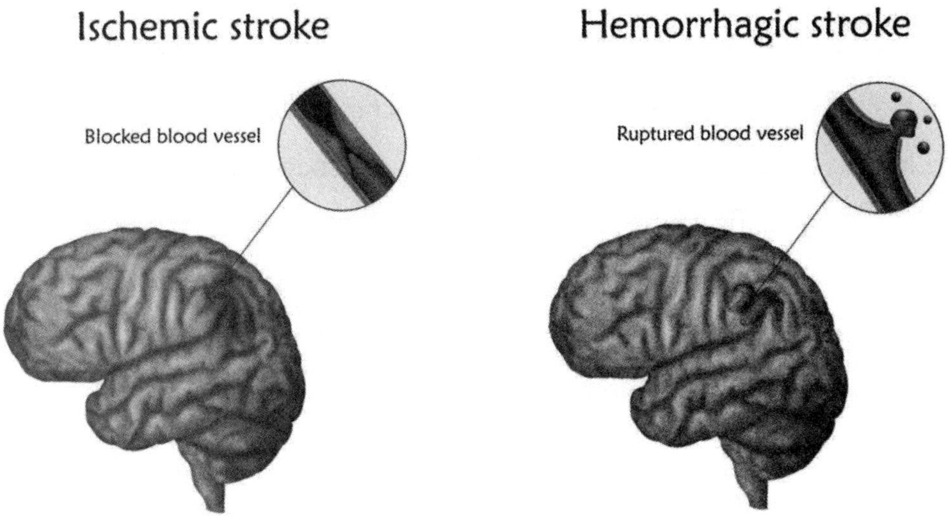

Stroke/Cerebrovascular Accident (CVA)

A **cerebrovascular accident (CVA)** occurs when the **blood supply** to a part of the **brain** is **interrupted** or **severely reduced,** depriving brain tissue of **oxygen** and **nutrients.** There are two primary types:

<u>Ischemic:</u> arteries to the brain become narrowed or blocked, causing severely reduced blood flow

<u>Hemorrhagic:</u> blood vessel in the brain leaks or ruptures.

A stroke can cause temporary or permanent disabilities depending on how long the brain lacks blood flow, and which part was affected. Common disabilities are paralysis, difficulty walking, difficulty talking or swallowing, memory loss/thinking difficulties, emotional problems, and pain.

Cochrane Reviews are systematic reviews of primary research in human health care and health policy, and are internationally recognized as the highest standard in evidence-based health care.

A **Cochrane Review** on acupuncture for stroke rehabilitation was completed in 2016. After reviewing all available medical research, the reviewers concluded: "From the available evidence, acupuncture may have beneficial effects on improving dependency, global neurological deficiency, and some specific neurological impairments for people with stroke in the convalescent stage, with no obvious serious adverse events" **("Acupuncture for Stroke Rehabilitation", Cochrane Database Sys Rev. 2016 August 26(8): CD004131). https://www.ncbi.nlm.nih.gov/pubmed/27562656**

Dive Deeper into Biomedicine- Acupuncture Promotes Functional Recovery in Stroke Patients

Stroke has been ranked as the **leading cause** of **motor disability** among adults across the world, which brings a **heavy burden** to the family and to society. **The ability to live independently after stroke depends largely on the recovery of motor function.**

In an interesting study using fMRI's of the brain, **acupuncture** was shown to **enhance** the **functional connectivity** between areas of the **brain** involved in **motor functions.** This means that acupuncture (at a point traditionally used for motor disorders) improved **neuroplasticity** (the brains ability to rewire itself) in response to a stroke **("Enhanced Functional Connectivity between the Bilateral Primary Motor Cortices after Acupuncture at *Yanglingquan* (GB34) in Right-Hemispheric Subcortical Stroke Patients: A Resting-State fMRI Study",** ***Front Hum Neurosci*** **2017 Apr 10; 11:178). https://www.ncbi.nlm.nih.gov/pubmed/28443010**

Another study showed "**acupuncture** may increase **motor-cognition connectivity** and decrease **compensation** of **unaffected motor cortex** and **homolateral synkinesis**, which can definitely **promote** the **rehabilitation** of **hemiplegia** and **spasm**" **("A Functional Magnetic Resonance Imaging Study on the Effect of Acupuncture at GB34 (*Yanglingquan*) on Motor-Related Network in Hemiplegic Patients",** ***Brain Res.*** **2015 Mar 19; 1601: 64-72). https://www.ncbi.nlm.nih.gov/pubmed/25601007**

Recommended Treatment Protocol: Physical Exam and twelve treatments (2x/week for 6 weeks) is considered one course of treatment. Multiple courses of treatment may be necessary. **It is best to start acupuncture sooner rather than later, because the efficacy of acupuncture for this condition depends on the severity and duration of symptoms.**

Treatment Goals: Improvement in functional abilities and ability to live independently.

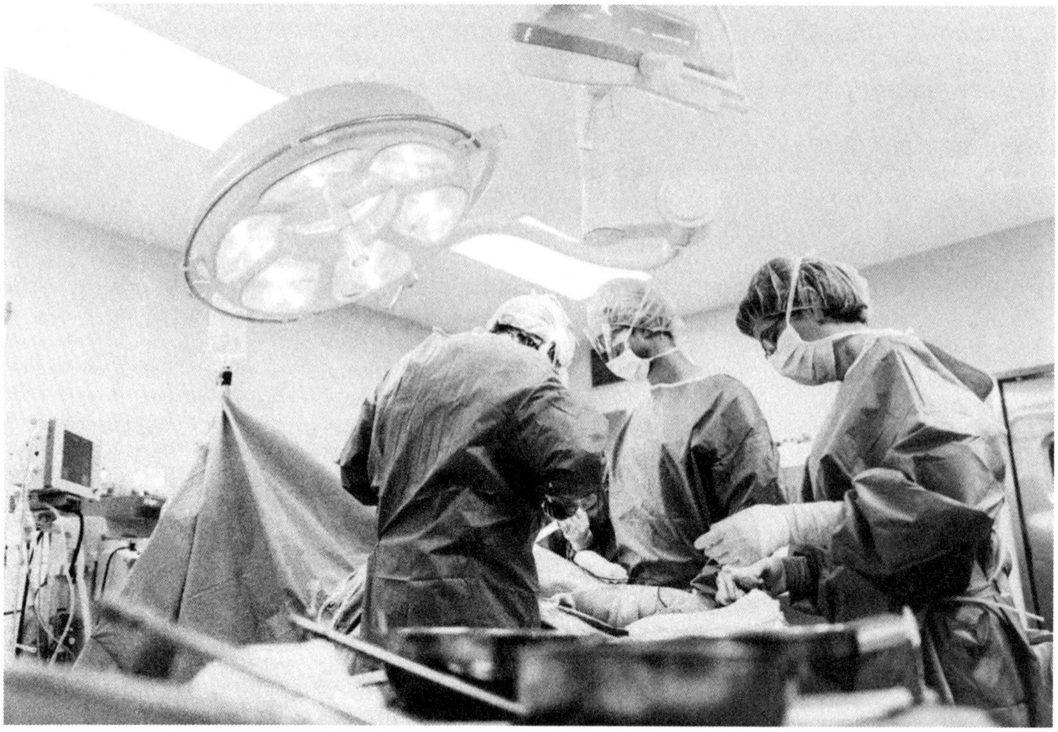

Surgery: General Recovery

People have **surgery** for many reasons- including **diagnostic**, **exploratory, plastic, corrective, elective,** and **life-saving** reasons. All **surgery**, by its very nature, is considered **acute trauma** to the body.

Acupuncture can play an important role in the **recovery process**. The administration of acupuncture immediately after surgery will greatly **reduce edema** and **swelling** and this accelerated fluid movement increases the **metabolism** of the **anesthetics** to increase the **elimination** of **remnant anesthetics** from the body.

Acupuncture will **speed healing** and promote **functional recovery**. Recent studies demonstrate that "acupuncture significantly improves **motor nerve conduction velocity** and **amplitude** and also promotes **functional nerve repair" (*Neural Regeneration Research* V10, no. 1 (2015): 128). https://www.ncbi.nlm.nih.gov/pmc/articles/PMC4357096/**

Further, **acupuncture** accelerates **recovery** after **general anesthesia ("Acupuncture Accelerates Recovery after General Anesthesia: A Prospective Randomized Controlled Trial",** ***J Integr Med.*** **2015 Mar; 13(2): 99-104).**
https://www.ncbi.nlm.nih.gov/pubmed/25797640

Acupuncture has also been traditionally used to reduce painful **scarring**. Recent studies have confirmed its effectiveness:

"The Successful Treatment of Pain Associated with Scar Tissue Using Acupuncture", ***JAMS*** **2014.05.001 http://www.sciencedirect.com/science/article/pii/S2005290114000922**

"Clinical Study on Treatment of Hypertonic Scar by Acupuncture", ***Research Gate*** **June 2011DOI: 10.1007.**
https://www.researchgate.net/publication/225747517_Clinical_study_on_treatment_of_hypertrophic_scar_by_acupuncture

Acupuncture can significantly **shorten** the **recovery process** and result in improved outcomes including the **reduction** of possible **complications.** It is best to start acupuncture as soon after the surgical procedure as realistically possible.

It is important to note that according to the **Centers for Disease Control (CDC),** smokers have a **lower survival rate** after surgery compared to that of nonsmokers because of **damage** to the **body's host defenses, delayed wound healing**, and **reduced immune response.** Smokers are at greater risk for **complications** following surgery, including **wound infections, postoperative pneumonia** and other **respiratory complications.**
https://www.cdc.gov/tobacco/data_statistics/sgr/2004/highlights/other_effects/index.htm . See **"Stop Smoking"** for more information on the importance of **quitting smoking** and how acupuncture can assist in this process.

Recommended Treatment Protocol: Physical Exam and eight treatments (2x/week for 4 weeks) is considered one course of treatment. Multiple courses of treatment may be necessary.

Treatment Goals: Speed healing and functional recovery, reduce scar formation and pain.

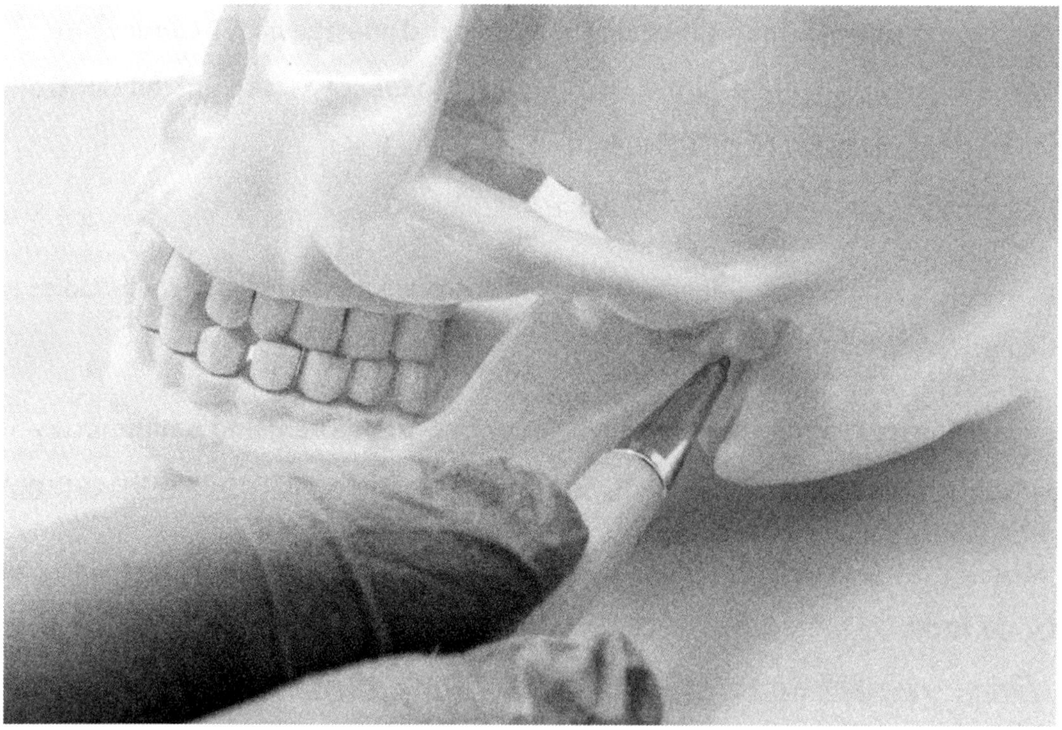

TMJ/TMD Recovery

The **temporomandibular joints (TMJ)** are the **hinge-like** joints that connect the **mandible** (lower jaw) to the **temporal bone** of the skull. The TMJ is susceptible to various disorders such as **inflammation, osteoarthritis,** or **rheumatoid arthritis**. **Pain** also may result from **mechanical damage** such as wear and tear on the joints, injury, tightened jaw muscles, stress, an improperly aligned bite, and poorly fitting braces or other dental appliances. Further, **chronic tension** and **anxiety** may cause a person to habitually **clench** the jaw or **grind** the teeth while sleeping. Once a person develops pain in the temporomandibular joint (TMJ), they are considered to have a **temporomandibular joint disorder (TMD)**.

A systematic review of all published medical literature regarding acupuncture for temporomandibular joint pain was completed in 2010. After analyzing all of the data, the researchers concluded: "This systematic review noted moderate evidence that **acupuncture** is an **effective intervention** to **reduce symptoms** associated with TMD" **("Acupuncture for Temporomandibular Disorders: A Systemic Review",** ***J Orofac Pain*** **2010 Spring; 24(2): 152-62). https://www.ncbi.nlm.nih.gov/pubmed/20401353**

Further, a study was done comparing acupuncture/deep dry needling to the standard drug therapy for TMJ pain. The researchers state "Acupuncture/deep dry needling of the trigger points in the LPM showed better efficacy in reducing pain and improving maximum mouth opening, laterality, and protrusion movements compared with drug treatment" **("Deep Dry Needling of Trigger Points Located in the Lateral Pterygoid Muscle: Efficacy and Safety of Treatment for Management of Myofascial Pain and Temporomandibular Dysfunction",** ***Med Oral Patol Oral Cir Bucal 2015*** **May 1; 20(3): e326-33). https://www.ncbi.nlm.nih.gov/pubmed/25662558**

Acupuncture can significantly **repair** injured **soft tissue** and restore **joint function.** It can also **slow** down the **degenerative process** in cases of **arthritis.** It is best to start acupuncture sooner rather than later, because the efficacy of acupuncture for this condition depends on the severity and duration of symptoms.

Recommended Treatment Protocol: Physical Exam and eight treatments (2x/week for 4 weeks) is considered one course of treatment. Multiple courses may be necessary. Maintenance treatment may be necessary.

Treatment Goals: Reduce the intensity, duration, and frequency of pain, reduce inflammation, reduce degeneration of the TM joint.

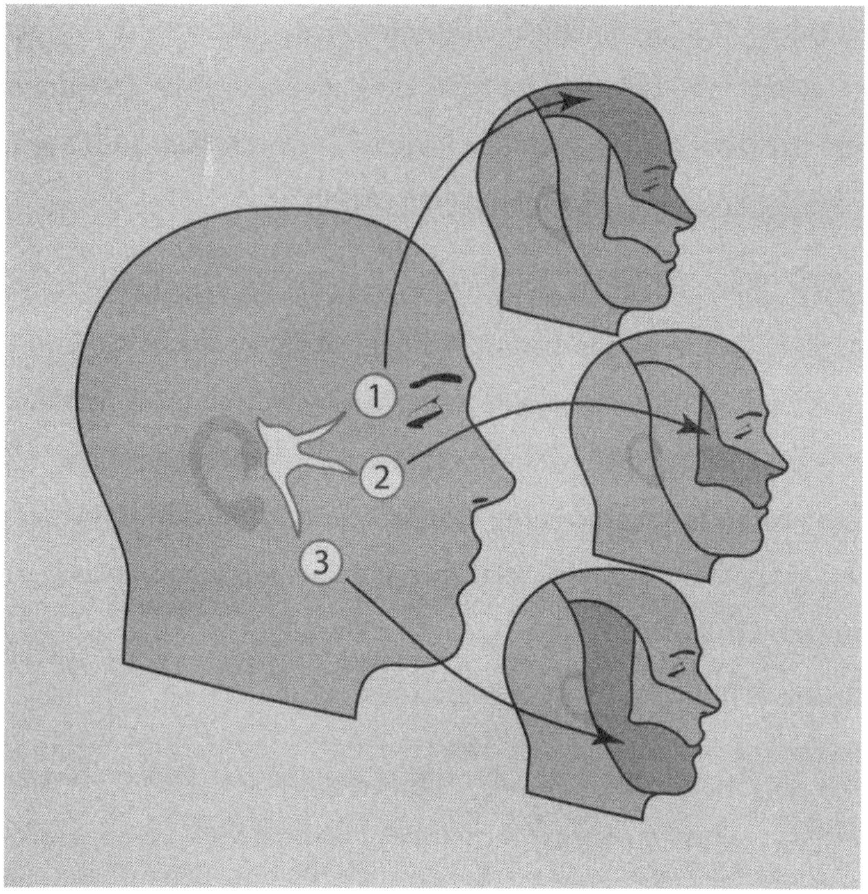

Trigeminal Neuralgia

Trigeminal Neuralgia (TN) is a chronic, recurring **pain** on **one side** of the **face**. The pain is caused by a disturbance in the function of the **trigeminal nerve**, which is the major nerve that carries the **sensation** from the **face** to the **brain**. The pain can be excruciating and may last for a few seconds or a few minutes. The exact **cause** is **unclear,** but is believed to involve the loss of **myelin** around the **trigeminal nerve**, possibly from **compression** from a **blood vessel**. TN is **medically managed** with either **drugs** or **surgery,** but both of these interventions may **not** be **effective** and may also cause unwanted **side effects** and other possible **complications**.

A review of all published medical literature regarding acupuncture for TN was conducted in 2010. Researchers found acupuncture was equal to standard drug therapy and concluded: "Acupuncture is of similar efficacy as carbamazepine but with fewer adverse effects" **("A Systematic Review of Acupuncture for Trigeminal Neuralgia",** ***Altern Ther Health Med.*** **2010 Nov-Dec; 16(6): 30-5). https://www.ncbi.nlm.nih.gov/pubmed/21280460**

Acupuncture can produce **excellent results** where other treatments fail. In one published case study, a patient had TN for 25 years and had tried **various treatments** (carbamazepine, trigeminal nerve block, and radiofrequency rhizotomy) but none adequately addressed her pain. After 14 acupuncture treatments (acupuncture three times per week for four weeks, twice per week for one week), she was completely **free of pain** and was still pain free at **six months** after treatment **("Successful Treatment of a Resistance Trigeminal Neuralgia Patient by Acupuncture",** ***Clinics (San Paulo)*** **2009 Dec; 64 (12): 1225-1226). https://www.ncbi.nlm.nih.gov/pmc/articles/PMC2797593/**

Acupuncture can significantly **shorten** the **recovery process** and result in a **significant reduction** in the **frequency** and **intensity** of TN **pain.** It is best to start acupuncture sooner rather than later, because the efficacy of acupuncture for this condition depends on the severity and duration of symptoms.

Recommended Treatment Protocol: Physical Exam and fourteen treatments (3x/week for 4 weeks, 2x/week for one week) is considered one course of treatment. Multiple courses may be necessary.

Treatment Goals: Reduce the intensity, duration, and/or frequency of TN pain.

NOTES

NOTES

NOTES

NOTES

NOTES

NOTES

NOTES